ARTHROSCOPY OF THE KNEE

MODERN ORTHOPEDIC MONOGRAPHS

Series Consultant
Robert E. Leach, M.D.
Boston University School of Medicine

Other books in the series
The Adolescent Spine   *Hugo A. Keim, M.D., F.A.C.S.*

ARTHROSCOPY OF THE KNEE

ROBERT W. JACKSON, M.D., M.S., F.R.C.S.(C)

Associate Professor
University of Toronto
Toronto, Canada

DAVID J. DANDY, F.R.C.S.

Consultant Orthopedic Surgeon
Addenbrooke's Hospital
Cambridge, England

GRUNE & STRATTON

A Subsidiary of Harcourt Brace Jovanovich, Publishers
New York   San Francisco   London

Library of Congress Cataloging in Publication Data

Jackson, Robert W
    Arthroscopy of the knee.

    (Modern orthopedic monographs)
    Bibliography: p.
    Includes index.
    1. Arthroscopy. 2. Knee—Diseases—Diagnosis.
I. Dandy, D. J., joint author. II. Title.
[DNLM: 1. Endoscopy. 2. Knee joint. WE870 J13a]
RC932.J3   617$'$.582$'$075   76-18916
ISBN 0-8089-0947-9

Grune & Stratton, Inc.
111 Fifth Avenue
New York, New York 10003

Distributed in the United Kingdom by
Academic Press, Inc. (London) Ltd.
24/28 Oval Road, London NW1

Library of Congress Catalog Number 76-18916
International Standard Book Number 0-8089-0947-9
Printed in the United States of America

TO MASAKI WATANABE

CONTENTS

FOREWORD

It seems strange that arthroscopy, which has come to be regarded as one of the orthopedist's and rheumatologist's most valuable tools, had such a long and painful birth, but such is the case.

One half a century ago, investigators such as Takagi in Japan, Bircher in Germany, and Burman in the United States reported some success in their efforts to visualize the interior of the knee with a scope, first a cystoscope and later an arthroscope. Their tools, however, were inadequate and, after a few reports from each country, the literature was silent. In 1960, Watanabe in Japan, undaunted by earlier failures, developed a first-class arthroscope complete with camera capable of producing sharp, clear, colored photographs of the interior of the knee.

By the mid 60's, a few physicians in the Western world, orthopedists and rheumatologists, essentially self-taught (as Watanabe and Japan were too far away), were attempting to arthroscope patients. Results of these endeavors began to appear in the orthopedic literature in the early 70's, and perhaps not surprisingly, these reports were received with skepticism and indifference. In the past two years, the value of a highly accurate diagnostic procedure which carries with it virtually no morbidity has finally been recognized, there has been a great surge of interest, and the manufacturers of the various instruments can scarcely keep pace with the demand.

There is certainly no one more qualified to write a book on the subject of arthroscopy than Bob Jackson, ably assisted by David Dandy. Dr. Jackson was introduced to arthroscopy by Watanabe in Japan, recognized its value, and in the past 10 years has acquired wide experience. He has documented and recorded his observations like the true scientist that he is and has established himself as the "Father of Arthroscopy in North America".

S. Ward Casscells, M.D.

ACKNOWLEDGMENTS

The significant assistance of the following is gratefully acknowledged: Miss Jan Godfrey—for the onerous task of preparing the manuscript; Professor F. P. Dewar—for encouraging and fostering our efforts in this field; Miss Margot Mackay—for illustrations; Mr. Richard Mikolajski of the Department of Medical Photography, Toronto General Hospital—for photographic assistance; the numerous anonymous patients—who provided the necessary experience; our colleagues and publishers—for their patience and forebearance; and particularly our wives and families without whose support and understanding this could never have been accomplished.

PREFACE

Historically, the *art* of medicine slowly and consistently converts to the *science* of medicine. With the advent of arthroscopy much of the guesswork about diagnosis and treatment of problems related to the knee joint has been eliminated. Indeed, good clinicians become even better, having mastered the technique of arthroscopy. For what is seen is what really exists. No longer does one have to rely on bits of information gathered under the heading of symptoms and signs, which may often be caused by any one of a variety of different disorders within the joint. Nor does one have to rely on the interpretation of shadows as created by plain x-rays or by arthrography, or have to resort to an exploratory arthrotomy to make or confirm a diagnosis. Although arthroscopy is an invasive diagnostic technique, its morbidity is so minimal, and its usefulness so great, that the technique is rapidly gaining increased usage throughout the world.

This book is an attempt to record our experiences, to outline the history and technique of the examination in some detail, and to describe normal and pathological conditions in a way that might prove useful to the practicing arthroscopist. It is not intended as a comprehensive atlas of knee joint pathology. Nor is it intended as a technical journal concerning instrumentation, as the tools of the technique are constantly changing with the rapid technology of our age. Having encountered most of the problems that can arise we also describe how to avoid them. We hardly need stress the tremendous potential for research into the physiology and pathology of joints.

It is our hope that this monograph will contribute to the overall management of knee problems by encouraging those who had previously ''opened the door widely'' to ''peek through the keyhole'' first, and by so doing to avoid intruding on intraarticular situations where such a surgical intrusion has little to offer.

Our personal thanks go to Dr. Masaki Watanabe to whom this book is gratefully dedicated and to his colleagues at the Tokyo Teishin Hospital who have so unselfishly promoted the technique of arthroscopy around the world. Our love and appreciation is also extended to our wives, Marilyn and Jane, and to both our families, for their understanding and support during the preparation of this book. We hope it will prove useful.

"From inability to let well alone;
From too much zeal for the new and
contempt for what is old;
From putting knowledge before wisdom,
science before art, and cleverness
before common sense;
From treating patients as cases, and
from making the cure of the disease
more grieveous than the endurance
of the same,
Good lord, deliver us."

Sir Robert Hutchinson
Modern Treatment, 1953

ARTHROSCOPY OF THE KNEE

1

The History of Arthroscopy

BACKGROUND OF ENDOSCOPY

The search for diagnostic certitude has led physicians to the endoscopic exploration of almost all of the previously sacrosanct body cavities. Yet the history of endoscopy is less than 200 years old. In the beginning, the problems were twofold: (1) how to introduce light into a body cavity to illuminate the structures within, and (2) once lit, how to see them.

Most historians attribute the beginning of endoscopy to Phillip Bozzini (1773–1809), who in 1806 presented his *lichtleiter* to the assembled members of the Joseph Academy of Medical Surgery in Vienna. The original instrument is long lost, but the apparatus reflected the light of a candle into a body cavity by means of several specula. Through the back of the instrument, there was a small opening, so that the cavity could be visualized. Although the principle of the experiment was appreciated, the members of the academy did not accept the *lichtleiter* and condemned it as a toy.

A few years later, Pierre S. Ségalas (1792–1875) used the same principle of light conduction to inspect the urethra and bladder. He demonstrated his instrument to the Royal French Academy, but the illumination it provided was minimal, and he failed to interest most of the surgeons in attendance.

A.J. Desormeaux (1815–1882) introduced the "cystoscope" in 1853. He developed a light source called a gazogene lamp, which used a mixture of turpentine and alcohol. The light generated by this lamp was then reflected into the bladder by a series of silver tubes and mirrors. A small opening in the center of a mirror enabled him to visualize the mucous membranes of the bladder. Improvements in instrumentation soon followed, but these new developments

1

were largely concerned with transmitting light more effectively from an external source to the interior of the bladder.

The next major advance came in 1876 when Max Nitze (1848–1906) introduced a light source *into* the bladder cavity. Nitze developed an instrument that used a heated platinum wire filament near the end of a tube that also contained reflectors. His main problem was that the lamp was extremely hot and had to be cooled. He was apparently heavily criticized for his "fire and water" invention.

Meanwhile, on the other side of the Atlantic Ocean, another invention was being perfected which proved to be a milestone in the development of endoscopy. In 1880, Edison introduced his incandescent lamp, a filament in a glass bulb, and in 1886, both Leopold Van Dittel (1815–1898) and Nitze incorporated the Edison lamp (called the Mignon lamp) into the cystoscope.

Shortly after this significant advance, Nitze also introduced the telescope principle to enlarge the field of vision, and in 1890 Nitze produced the first photocystoscope. R. Kutner took the first endoscopic photographs in that year.

Improvements in lighting and optics then followed in rapid succession. In 1907, the Zeiss Company improved their optical system by using a combination of lenses in a different type of prism (the Amici prism). This produced a vertical and sharper image which was also much brighter because less light was lost in transmission. Before this, the image was always inverted.

ARTHROSCOPY

Professor K. Takagi (1883–1963) of Tokyo University was the first to explore the interior of a human knee joint in 1918 (Fig. 1-1). He used a cystoscope, Charrière number 22, and from this experience he began to design an endoscopic instrument particularly suitable for inspecting joint cavities. The first "arthroscope" Takagi designed was 7.3 mm in diameter and contained no lens system; however, it had an incandescent bulb at the tip. Because it involved direct visualization down a narrow tube, the field of vision was very small. Moreover, the large diameter of the scope made it relatively impractical for use in human knee joints. Takagi therefore concentrated on reducing the diameter of the scope and made a series of models with progressively smaller diameters. By 1931, he had reduced the diameter to 3.5 mm. Subsequent models were even smaller; number 11 had a diameter of 2.7 mm and was designed for use in the canine knee. With the smaller scopes, a lens system was needed to magnify the images seen.

The original impetus for this work was a desire to diagnose tuberculosis of the knee joint in its earliest stages, and possibly therefore to influence treatment. The end result of the tuberculous knee was frequently an ankylosed joint, and the inability to bend the knee was a serious social as well as physical disability in Japan.

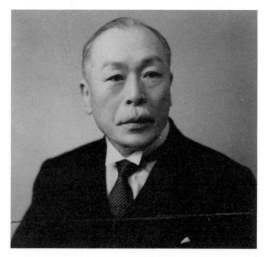

Fig. 1-1. Kenji Takagi (1883–1963), Professor of
Orthopedics, University of Tokyo. The first man to
adapt endoscopy to the knee joint (1918).

Takagi's next scope, the number 12, was 4 mm in diameter; this slightly
larger, more robust scope enabled the surgeon to perform biopsies under direct
vision. His number 13 introduced forward oblique and side viewing lenses for
the first time. Takagi developed the number 14 scope in the mid 1930s, and this
instrument (which was 5 mm in diameter and had a straight ahead lens system)
was used in 1936 to take the first color photographs of the inside of a knee joint.
The photographs were obtained using an additional light source through a
second insertion (Fig. 1-2).

Professor Takagi's talented pupil and successor was Dr. Masaki
Watanabe (Fig. 1-3), who continued to develop new arthroscopes when optical
and electronic technology was becoming one of the major industries of Japan.
Dr. Watanabe also continued the consecutive numbering system for each new
scope.

The number 19 "Watanabe" arthroscope proved extremely practical and
was widely used in his clinic for several years.

The first *Atlas of Arthroscopy* was published by Watanabe in 1957 and
was illustrated by intra-articular views painted by Mr. S. Fujihashi.

Another major advance came in 1959 when the number 21 arthroscope
was developed. This instrument had a sheath 6.5 mm in diameter, a straight
ahead view wide angle lens that provided a field of vision of 102°, and an
excellent tungsten light source at the tip. For almost 10 years, this instrument
has been the instrument of choice for arthroscopists around the world. Excellent photographs can be obtained using the number 21 scope.

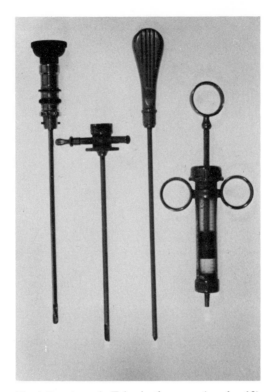

Fig. 1-2.   An early Takagi arthroscope (number 13),
1932.

In Watanabe's number 22 scope, developed in 1967, fiber light is used for illumination at the expense of a slightly reduced field of vision.

Watanabe's number 23 scope was a prototype fiber optic scope 2 mm in diameter which was rapidly improved with models 24 and 25.

As is often the case, another pioneer on the other side of the world to Takagi was at the same time, and quite independently, exploring endoscopic applications to the human knee joint. In 1921 Professor E. Bircher (1882–1956) (Fig. 1–4) in Switzerland reported his experience in "Arthroendoscopy". In 1922, using a Jacobeus laparoscope built by George Wolf of Berlin and a technique that involved distending the knee joint with oxygen and nitrogen (using an artificial pneumothorax apparatus), Bircher reported his findings in 20 cases of traumatic osteoarthritis. It is of clinical interest that he commented, almost in passing, that insured patients did not get well as quickly as those who did not have insurance.

In 1924 Philip H. Kreuscher (1884–1943) presented to the Illinois Medical Society a paper that was published in the Illinois Medical Journal in 1925.

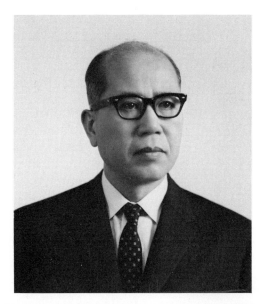

Fig. 1-3. Masaki Watanabe, current Professor of Orthopedics, Tokyo Teishin Hospital. Takagi's successor and pioneer in developing modern arthroscopes and techniques.

His topic was semilunar cartilage disease, and he pleaded for the early recognition of meniscal damage by means of the arthroscope. Unfortunately, his paper gave no details about the arthroscope that he developed and used, although it provided a picture of the instrument.

In the early 1930s, Dr. Michael Burman (1901–1975) at the Hospital for Joint Diseases in New York City began his studies on arthroscopy. In a classic article published in October 1931, Burman described his work to that date using an arthroscope constructed by Mr. R. Wappler. The trocar was 4 mm in diameter, and the telescope was 3 mm in diameter. A constant irrigation system was used.

Using this instrument, Burman explored all possible approaches to the knee joint and also explored arthroscopic applications in other joints. The instrumentation of that time, however, was not robust and occasionally he had problems with the light source. Thus, Burman's colleagues only partly appreciated his work.

Drs. L. Mayer, H. Finkelstein, and C.J. Sutro, at the same hospital, also explored possible applications of endoscopy to synovial joints, and over the next 8 years they were responsible with Dr. Burman for several significant articles on the subject.

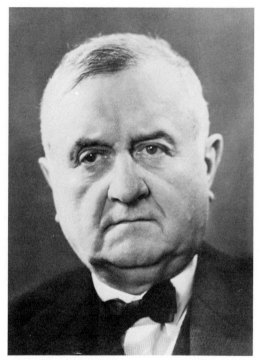

Fig. 1-4. Eugen Bircher (1882–1956), Aarau, Switzerland, developed his own technique of arthroendoscopy using a Jacobeus laparoscope and was the first person to publish an article on the subject.

In 1937 and 1938, articles by Drs. R. Sommer and E. Vaubel were published in the German literature.

Over the next few years, possibly because of the martial turmoil in the world at that time, there was a noticeable hiatus in publications on the subject, although Dr. F. Koike in 1943 and Dr. T. Okamura in 1945 published articles in the Japanese literature. Perhaps also the technology of that time was still insufficient to permit adequate and useful application of the technique to joints.

In 1955 E. Hurter, writing in French, described a "new" method of examining joints by an arthroscope, and in 1956 and 1957 R. Imbert also published articles in French on the significance and technique of arthroscopy. In 1960 R. Suckert wrote in German about photoarthroscopy of the knee joint.

In 1960 the Watanabe number 21 arthroscope was made available for general use, and in 1967 J. Robles-Gil and G. Katona in Mexico published articles on the use of this instrument in studies of rheumatoid joints.

In 1964 the senior author of this book lived in Tokyo while working in the Department of Anatomy at Tokyo University. He heard about the work of Dr. Watanabe but was extremely skeptical. His first reaction on seeing the interior of a joint with such clarity was typical of everyone who has also had this opportunity: enthusiasm and appreciation for what the future might hold through applying this technique to the study of joint disease and trauma. Dr. Watanabe and his colleagues Dr. H. Ikeuchi and Dr. S. Takeda taught the author as much as they could about arthroscopy, and on returning to Canada in 1965, the author in turn taught others and revived interest in the technique in North America.

Since that time, many individuals—including Drs. Jayson, Dixon, Ohnsorge, Dorfmann, Dreyfuss, Casscells, O'Connor, Joyce, Johnson, Eikelaar, and many others—have made significant contributions to the field of arthroscopy. These and other interested arthroscopists from around the world formed the International Arthroscopy Association in Philadelphia in 1974, with this objective: "to foster by means of arthroscopy the development and dissemination of knowledge in the fields of orthopedics and medicine in order to improve the diagnosis and treatment of joint disorders." Dr. Masaki Watanabe was elected the first president.

2

Equipment

Like other endoscopic instruments, the arthroscope consists essentially of three components: an optical system, a lighting system, and an irrigation system. As these may vary considerably in design and characteristics from one model of arthroscope to the next, we feel it is useful, for both the beginner and the experienced arthroscopist, to know the potentials of the individual instruments. In this chapter, we describe the characteristics of the different instruments that are currently available, rather than compare the benefits of one design with those of another.

OPTICAL SYSTEM

The *field of vision* of the arthroscope is conical with the apex at the lens. This cone may be broader or narrower in angle according to the optical design. The broader the angle of vision, the easier it is for the arthroscopist to orient himself within the knee. On the other hand, the design and manufacture of the lenses necessary for wide angle vision are technically more difficult.

The *angle of vision* quoted for a lens should be stated as either in normal saline or in air, as the angle of vision in air is far greater. Figure 2-1 shows the practical difference between angles of vision of 100°, 90°, 70°, and 55°. A wide angle of vision is easier to obtain if the instrument has a large diameter, but a large diameter limits the mobility and usefulness of the instrument within the knee. A narrow telescope with a comparatively smaller angle of vision may reach recesses at the back of the joint that are inaccessible to a larger instrument, so the former may be more useful in tighter knees.

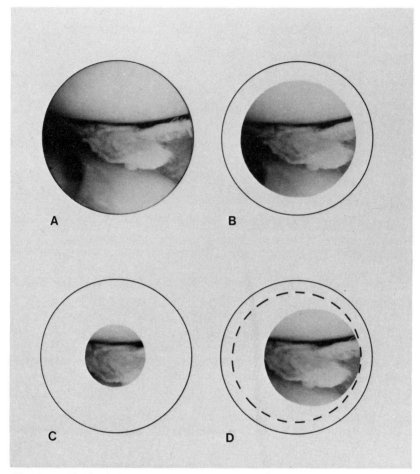

Fig. 2-1.   Fields of vision possible with various angles of vision.
A. 100°; *B.* 90°; *C.* 55°; *D.* 70°. With a fore-oblique lens, rotating the scope allows a larger area to be visualized (*dotted line*).

The field of vision may extend directly ahead from the end of the arthroscope or may deviate up to 90° from the long axis of the instrument. Such a 90°-instrument is available with the Watanabe 21 arthroscope and is useful for looking around corners and at the undersurface of the patella. However, its use is limited by problems in orientation. With other instruments, the field of vision is only slightly deviated to one side of the midline. As the field of vision is still essentially forward, although slightly oblique, these instruments are described as "forward-oblique" or "fore-oblique" scopes, and the direction of vision is recorded as the angle between a line drawn from the midpoint of the field of vision and a line along the shaft of the instrument. To avoid confusion, we prefer to use the terms "angle of vision" to denote the extent of the visual field and "direction of vision" to indicate the angle at which the visual field is directed—straight ahead being 0° (Fig. 2-2).

When the direction of vision is not straight ahead, the operator can increase the field of vision by turning the arthroscope 360° around its long axis, sweeping the field much like the beam from a lighthouse (Fig. 2-1d). Orienta-

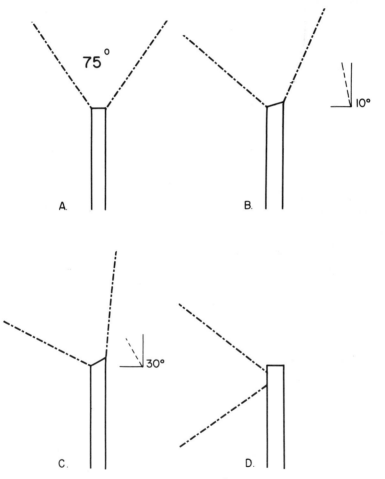

Fig. 2-2.   The angle of vision in each instance is 75°, but the direction of vision varies. *A*. 0° or straight ahead; *B*. 10° fore-oblique; *C*. 30° fore-oblique; *D*. 90° side view.

tion is not lost because the portion of the field directly ahead remains in view as the instrument is turned.

The image that is seen is transmitted to the eye by one of several optical measures. One method, such as that used in the Watanabe 21 and Wolf arthroscopes, employs a series of conventional glass lenses contained within a rigid tube. The Storz instruments use the Hopkins lens system, which consists of air spaces between glass rods, the ends of which are shaped so that the air spaces act as the lenses. With this system, distortion due to slight bending of the telescope causes a dark crescent to appear at one edge of the field of vision ("vignetting"). Far from being a disadvantage, this distortion encourages gentleness by providing visual feedback when excessive force is being applied to the instrument.

Most of the small scopes use a single glass fiber 1.7 mm in diameter that is specially coated to provide good image transmission over a significant distance.* The image received at the proximal end of the glass fiber is then magnified by conventional lenses for easy viewing. This is basically the method used in the Dyonics Needlescope, the Watanabe 25 arthroscope, and the Olympus Selfoscope. A fourth method of image transmission, which is widely employed in the flexible endoscopes used to explore other body cavities, consists of a bundle of optical glass fibers, each fiber transmitting a portion of the visual field. At the time of this writing, the resolution or visual clarity obtained by this system is markedly inferior to that achieved with the other methods, so the system is not used. However, in this era of rapid technological advancement, a flexible arthroscope is a definite possibility for the future.

Accessories to prevent unsterile eyelashes and eyebrows from touching the eyepiece of the arthroscope are available (e.g., sterile eyeglasses, sterile masks, hoods, shields, etc.; Fig. 2-3), but most users prefer simply to keep their eye about 1 inch from the eyepiece, a technique that is not difficult with practice.

The depth of focus in most instruments is from 1–2 mm to infinity. In practice, objects less than 2 mm from the lens appear so enormous through magnification that it is almost impossible to appreciate them.

The lens systems magnify the image by an amount that is constant for each instrument. This is of some practical importance because the proximity of the object to the lens has a greater effect on the magnification than the design of the lens system. With the Watanabe number 21 lens, an object 1 mm from the lens is magnified 10 times, at 1 cm it is magnified 2 times, and at 2 cm from the lens it appears its normal size. In all endoscopes, the magnification of an object generally varies as the inverse ratio of its distance from the tip.

---

*Trademark *Selfoc.*

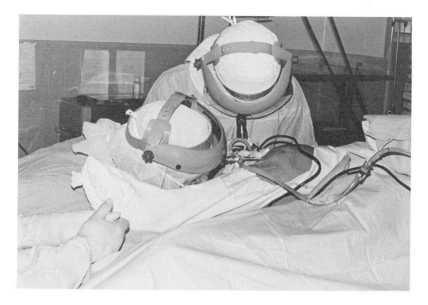

Fig. 2-3.   Sterile accessories are available to maintain aseptic technique (courtesy Dr. R.C. Bechtol).

LIGHTING SYSTEM

The two major ways of illuminating the inside of the knee are with a tungsten light bulb, as used by the Watanabe 21 (Fig. 2-4), or with fiber light, as used by the Watanabe 22 (Fig. 2-5) and all of the other major arthroscopes. Although problems occur with the tungsten bulb (bending and breaking have been reported with rough handling), it provides good light for visualization and easy photography. Two other minor problems are the heat produced by the bulb and the occasional electrical short circuit.

Fiber light systems are designed so that the fiber light cable is an integral part of the instrument or it can be detached.

One disadvantage of a cable that detaches from the instrument is light loss. When the fibers end and rejoin a certain amount of light is lost, and the advantages of a separate cable must be weighed against this. A further disadvantage is that some fibers in the cable may break due to kinking or bending, permanently reducing brilliance; but this possibility can be minimized by careful handling of the cable and in particular by never twisting or coiling the cable tightly. The light that is delivered to the end of the arthroscope is proportional to the number of fibers passing down the scope and the intensity of the light source. The larger the arthroscope, the more light that can be made available; but again, this advantage must be weighed against the problem of increasing bulk.

Adapters are easily made to connect any fiber light cable to any existing fiber light source.

Fiber light systems, in which glass fibers transmit light down the scope, must be distinguished from fiber optic systems, in which the glass fibers carry the optical image up the scope to the eye. Some of the smaller arthroscopes, particularly the Watanabe 25 and the Dyonics Needlescope, use a fiber optic system to carry the image from inside the joint to the ocular lens system outside, which magnifies the image. In most instances, however, the resolution that can be obtained with lens systems is technically superior to that obtained by fiber optic systems.

If photographs are to be taken, a flash generator or capacitor may be necessary. These are components of the fiber light source and can raise the brilliance of the light for a fraction of a second while a photograph is taken. The Watanabe 21, which has a tungsten bulb, has a second electrical circuit by which the voltage can be doubled temporarily to make the bulb burn brighter, allowing photographs to be taken. If light for photography is minimal, the developing and processing of some films can be "forced" so that photographs can be taken without special flash equipment; however, the quality of such photographs may suffer as a result. Daylight film is used with fiber light sytems, and type "B" film is used with the tungsten (incandescent) light system. In the future, faster color films will undoubtedly be developed, or methods of electronic amplification and videotape recording will evolve that will minimize the light problem.

IRRIGATION SYSTEM

Some arthroscopes, particularly those with small diameters, do not allow for continuous irrigation during examination. A tourniquet is applied and the joint is inflated with saline under some pressure so that bleeding is kept to a minimum. This allows excellent conditions for the examination, but in our opinion, the tourniquet-imposed anemia makes it difficult to detect minor changes in the vascularity of the synovium and sometimes to differentiate between degenerative articular cartilage and synovial fronds.

If the tourniquet is not inflated, the natural colors of the tissues are preserved. However, minor bleeding may obscure vision in the absence of a current of saline, and for this reason we prefer continuous irrigation. In a constant stream of saline, blood is washed away, synovial fronds and fibrillated articular cartilage move in the stream of saline, and the pathological features are delineated more clearly.

We prefer normal saline at room temperature as an irrigating solution.

SIZE OF THE INSTRUMENT

Arthroscopes vary in their outside diameter from 2–6.5 mm. Although a small instrument of 2 mm in diameter can penetrate to the deepest recesses of the knee, it can also be broken easily if the knee is flexed or unwarranted force is applied. On the other hand, a larger instrument is more robust and provides better optics, brighter light, and a larger sheath for inserting operating instruments, even though it may be too large to explore all areas of the joint.

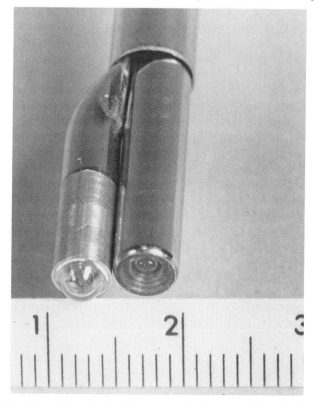

Fig. 2-4.   Watanabe 21. The tungsten light bulb is offset and lying alongside the arthroscope. With care, it can be used for retracting synovial fronds.

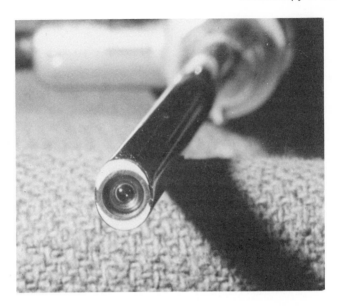

Fig. 2-5. Watanabe 22. The light fibers for illumination are grouped into 2 crescentic bundles on either side of the arthroscope, which eliminates a penumbra in the center of the visual field.

In practice, each of the instruments available has certain advantages and certain limitations, which can be discussed incessantly. The accomplished arthroscopist should have a variety of scopes available to meet the variety of clinical problems that will arise.

The Watanabe 21 has a 6.5-mm cannula, but the tungsten light bulb is offset so that the tip of the instrument is 10 mm by 5 mm (Fig. 2-4). The offset bulb provides an advantage in that it can be used as a sweeper or retractor to move fronds of synovium out of the visual field.

The Watanabe 22 arthroscope uses the same sheath (6.5 mm) but adds fiber light to the scope at the expense of some angle of vision.

The Richard Wolf arthroscope also has a 6.5-mm cannula through which two sizes of telescopes are inserted. The 5-mm telescope is used for photography and diagnosis; the 2.5-mm telescope leaves enough room for inserting operating tools down the same sheath while providing enough vision to permit accurate biopsy. Alternatively, the 2.5-mm scope can be used with a 4-mm cannula.

The Storz arthroscope has 3.5- and 4.5-mm sheaths, whereas the Dyonics and the Watanabe 25 have a 2-mm cannula.

ACCESSORIES

Many accessories are available for these arthroscopes. Most manufacturers supply biopsy forceps that are passed down the barrel of the operating instrument or through a separate incision. The advantage of passing forceps directly down the barrel is that the tip of the forceps is always directly in front of the lens (Fig. 2-6). If the instrument is passed through a separate cannula from the other side of the knee, the tip of the instrument may be surprisingly difficult to locate visually. Inserting instruments through a separate cannula requires three hands: one to manipulate the arthroscope, another to manipulate the instrument, and a third to manipulate the leg. Therefore, a good assistant is essential.

Biopsy forceps are naturally intended for obtaining synovial biopsies, but they are also useful in catching loose bodies as they slip and slide within the joint (Fig. 2-7).

Operating scissors that are passed through a separate cannula are also

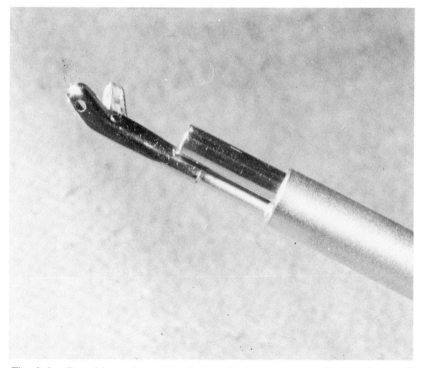

Fig. 2-6. Storz biopsy forceps can be passed down the same sheath with a small diameter arthroscope, permitting biopsy under direct vision.

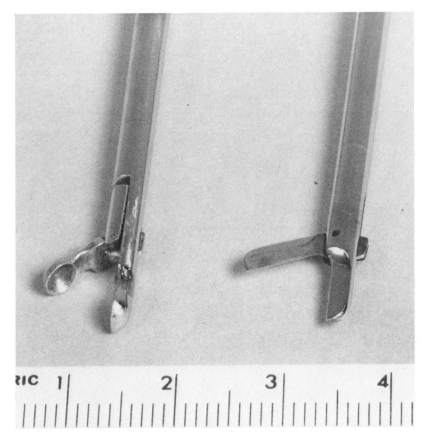

Fig. 2-7. Watanabe forceps and operating scissors can be inserted through a second sheath, permitting some intra-articular surgery to be carried out under direct vision.

available with some scopes. These are particularly useful for intra-articular surgery (Fig. 2-7).

Teaching attachments, using beam splitters (which divert an image of lesser light intensity to an assistant or observer), are useful for teaching or for attempting surgical procedures through the scope when an extra pair of hands is essential. In the future, videotapes will probably provide the most useful teaching aid.

CAMERAS

Most camera bodies can be adapted to fit the arthroscope, and all the manufacturers can supply a suitable modified camera for their instrument. A single-lens reflex camera that takes 35-mm film is preferable. Full-frame or half-frame cameras are available.

Cinephotography and television are also possible, but they often require more light than is available with the present equipment.

STERILIZATION

It is important to know what method of sterilization may be safe with the different types of arthroscopes. All the existing arthroscopes can be gas sterilized safely with carboxicide (88 percent) and ethylene oxide (12 percent) for the usual 4-hour cycle at 71°C in a gas autoclave. Most can be sterilized in antiseptic solution by soaking for an appropriate period of time (e.g., 1/750 Detergicide solution for 20 minutes), and formalin vapor sterilization is still used in Japan. The Storz and Wolf arthroscopes can be sterilized in an autoclave if the manufacturers' instructions are followed carefully.

A quick method of sterilization is important to permit treatment of patients consecutively. Otherwise, more than one arthroscope should be available.

3
The Normal Examination

If one is appropriately selective in choosing cases for arthroscopy and appropriately perceptive in detecting pathological conditions, the number of truly "normal" examinations will be minimal. However, as a high-spirited minister once said, "You must know sin, to preach against it." Similarly, you must know the normal anatomy in order to appreciate the sometimes subtle pathological changes that might be encountered.

In this chapter we will describe in some detail our technique and the normal appearance of each area of the knee that is visualized.

The basic technique is that of Watanabe modified only slightly by the authors. Further modifications also make the technique suitable for fiber light scopes.

First of all, as in any invasive diagnostic procedure, there is a risk of contamination; therefore, arthroscopy should be performed only in the operating room under aseptic conditions and with full sterile ritual.

ANESTHESIA

We prefer general anesthesia for three reasons: (1) if a lesion is found, it is quite easy to proceed to definitive treatment using the same anesthetic; (2) the patient feels no discomfort if the tourniquet is inflated; and (3) complete muscle relaxation is obtained, which permits a more thorough examination, including assessment of ligament stability, and eliminates any risk of inadvertent patient movement while the instrument is in the back of the joint.

However, local anesthetics can be effective in certain circumstances. Reexamination of the patellofemoral joint after shaving, examination or biopsy of synovium, and irrigation of the joint in known cases of crystal synovitis are specific indications for a local anesthetic. Other practical indications for a local anesthetic might exist, such as when hospital regulations require patients undergoing general anesthesia to be admitted the day before an operation or examination and remain in the hospital for at least one day afterwards.

If a local anesthetic is to be used, we recommend infiltration of the skin with Xylocaine 1 percent at the site of insertion or blocking of the infrapatellar branch of the saphenous nerve, followed by injection of 50 cc of normal saline containing 10 cc of Xylocaine 2 percent into the knee and left for 5 minutes before beginning the examination. We have found that this regime provides adequate relief of discomfort except when the tourniquet is inflated or the joint is stressed to open its posterior corners. The conscious patient should be warned that he may also notice a peculiar sensation when the synovium is pulled at the moment of biopsy.

Recently we have used "neurolept analgesia" plus small amounts of a local anesthetic with pleasing results.

Spinal or epidural anesthesia is also possible.

EXAMINATION UNDER ANESTHESIA

When the patient or the knee is anesthetized, the physician should examine the joint in this painless and relaxed condition before drapes and other constrictions are applied. It is important to test carefully for ligamentous and capsular instability and for any intra-articular clicks that may have been missed when the patient was awake. Examination under anesthesia in this way should not be omitted; it can yield more information about the integrity of the ligaments than arthroscopy.

TOURNIQUET APPLICATION

The tourniquet is applied to the upper thigh but usually is not inflated unless bleeding occurs that cannot be cleared by irrigation. If bleeding persistently obscures vision, the leg is elevated for 2 minutes to empty the veins passively, and the tourniquet is inflated. At the end of the examination, the tourniquet is released and the knee is repeatedly washed until all signs of blood have disappeared. This may require several hundred cubic centimeters of saline.

The advantage of examining the knee without the tourniquet inflated is that the synovium is seen in its normal color and its vascular nature can be evaluated. This is often important in determining whether the frondlike structures that are visualized are synovial in origin or are degenerative articular or meniscal cartilage. If an examination is performed totally under tourniquet control, the synovium pales quickly and it is often difficult to appreciate subtle changes in synovial appearance.

DRAPING THE LEG

The method of draping is a matter of personal preference, but two points deserve mention. First, there is always some leakage from the irrigation system which soaks the drapes and the table beneath. Because this is a potential pathway for infection if arthrotomy follows arthroscopy, we use a waterproof drape.

Second, the drapes around the lower leg should be as compact as possible so that they do not touch the surgeon's face or mask any more than necessary.

Apart from these two considerations, draping of the leg is unremarkable. We prepare the skin with iodine (Fig. 3-1). A green sheet is laid across the operating table, and a small towel is attached high up the thigh to cover the tourniquet (Fig. 3-2). A waterproof split sheet is then applied while an assistant

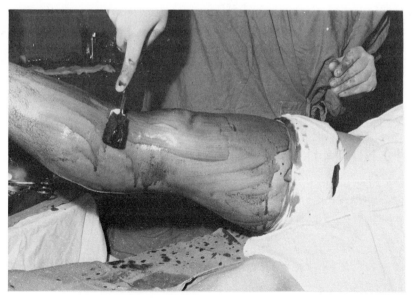

Fig. 3-1.   A full surgical preparation with the tourniquet in place but not inflated.

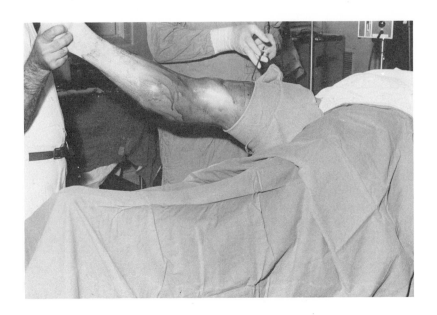

Fig. 3-2.   Application of sterile drapes.

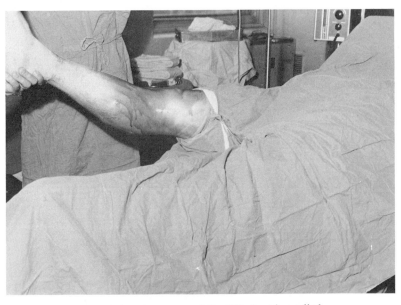

Fig. 3-3.   A waterproof "split" sheet is applied.

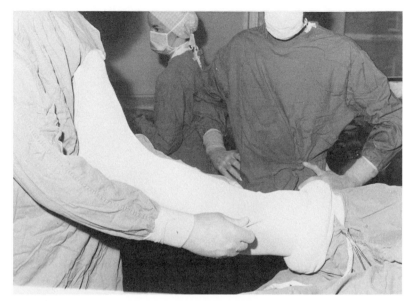

Fig. 3-4. Double-layer of stockinette is used to cover the foot and leg.

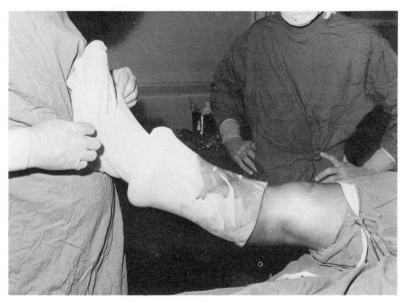

Fig. 3-5. The roll of stockinette is pulled down to minimize bulk of drapes just below the knee.

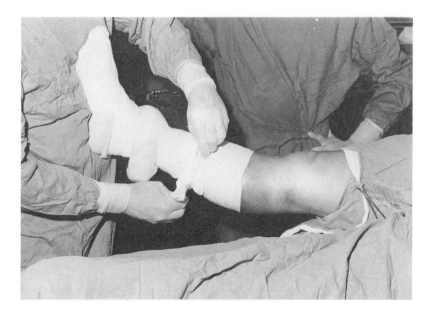

Fig. 3-6. The stockinette is tied with a roll of flannelette bandage to minimize the drapes, and secure the stockinette.

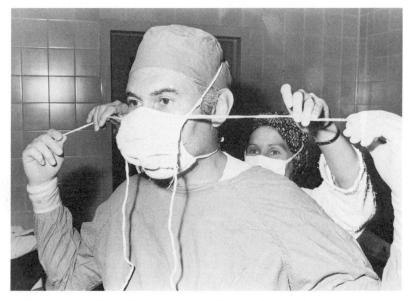

Fig. 3-7. A second sterile mask is donned.

26

holds the leg (Fig. 3-3), and a double thickness of stockinette is rolled up the leg to just above the knee (Fig. 3-4). The stockinette cuff is then pulled down over itself to the level of the ankle, leaving the inner layer about 4 inches below the knee (Fig. 3-5). The stockinette is tied to the leg tightly with a 4-inch flannel bandage with the knot placed on the medial side so that it does not get in the way of the examination, which is usually performed from the lateral approach (Fig. 3-6).

We use sterile masks routinely. An unsterile gauze mask is worn while the patient is prepared, and then an assistant applies a sterile mask over the first (Fig. 3-7).

ASPIRATION AND DISTENSION OF THE JOINT

The knee is aspirated with a 15- or 16-gauge needle inserted in the suprapatellar pouch at the superolateral corner of the patella (Fig. 3-8). The needle is left in situ to serve as an outflow tube for the irrigating solution and as a tool for palpating structures in the suprapatellar pouch and the undersurface of the patella.

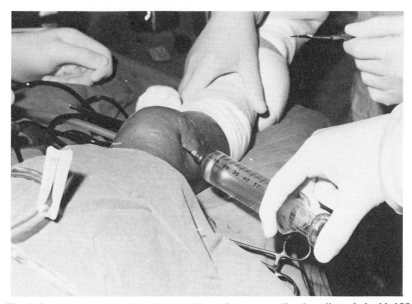

Fig. 3-8.   The knee joint is aspirated with a 16-gauge needle, then distended with 100 ml of normal saline at room temperature. The most common point of insertion is deep to the superolateral corner of the patella.

To insert the needle, the physician first fully extends the knee and displaces the patella laterally until he can feel the angle of the superolateral corner. The needle is directed distally at an angle of 45° to the long axis of the leg and kept parallel with the undersurface of the patella (being careful not to scrape the articular cartilage). An experienced physician can penetrate the joint and feel the articular cartilage in the patellofemoral compartment with the tip of the needle. The joint contents are then aspirated and kept for any laboratory examination that may be indicated. Then 75–100 cc of normal saline at room temperature is injected to distend the joint before inserting the arthroscope.

IRRIGATING SOLUTION

The irrigating solution of choice is normal saline at room temperature. If the saline is too cold, it tends to blanch the synovium and produce a relatively avascular appearance. Saline that is too warm causes hyperemia, which can be confused with an inflammatory reaction of the synovium. Normal saline is chosen because it is innocuous and appears to have no long-term adverse effects on articular cartilage or synovium. Glucose solutions have been used for their hemolytic effect, but we do not recommend them because they can have deleterious effects on the kidney. Although some arthroscopists use air or carbon dioxide to distend the joint, this is not commonly done since it tends to dry the structures of the knee, making early fibrillation of articular cartilage difficult to detect.

The irrigating solution of saline should be elevated approximately 1 meter above the knee, thus providing enough hydrostatic pressure to keep the joint distended (given the resistance of a 15-gauge outflow needle) and to maintain a current of irrigating fluid sufficient to wash away any blood or debris (Fig. 3-9).

INSERTION OF THE ARTHROSCOPE

Sites

The most common point of entry is anterolaterally at the joint line, as close to the patellar tendon and the upper surface of the tibia as possible without penetrating or passing beneath the meniscus or damaging the patellar tendon.

The position of insertion is best determined by flexing the knee to 45° and feeling for the upper border of the tibia with the tip of the thumb. Close to the lateral edge of the patellar tendon is a small fossa into which the thumb can be pressed (Fig. 3-10). When this has been identified, the thumb is pushed in as far as possible, keeping the distal phalanx parallel to the upper border of the tibial

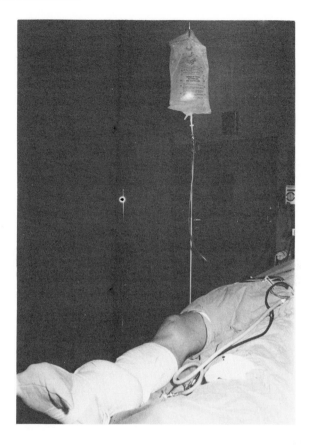

Fig. 3-9.   The joint is constantly irrigated due to hydrostatic pressure. The bag or bottle of saline is elevated 1 meter above the knee
joint, and the fluid drains through the instrument and out through the
needle in the suprapatellar pouch.

plateau. The surgeon must avoid pushing the skin up or pulling it down during
this procedure, or the insertion will be too high or too low, and the examination
will be very difficult.

A 4-mm skin incision is then made just above the thumb nail. A narrow
scalpel blade is suitable for this purpose. The incision should be just deep
enough to reach the capsule (Fig. 3-11).

The arthroscope may also be inserted either medial or lateral to the upper
pole of the patella or in the midline above it. These suprapatellar insertions are
useful for examining the patellofemoral compartment and the suprapatellar
pouch, but they are of little use for inspecting the menisci.

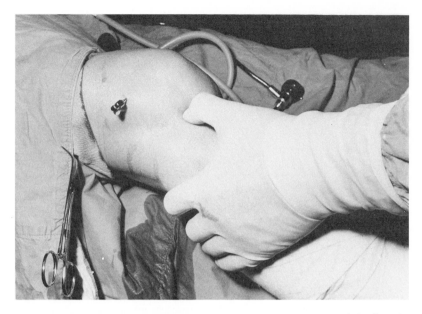

Fig. 3-10.   The most common point of insertion is anteriorly, at the joint line, just lateral to the patellar tendon (see text).

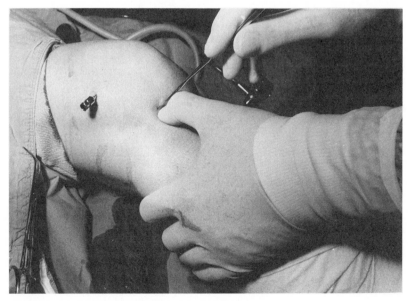

Fig. 3-11.   A 4-mm stab incision is made down to capsule, just above the nail of the palpating thumb.

30

If need be, the arthroscope can be inserted posteromedially, allowing this somewhat difficult area to be inspected directly.

Technique of Insertion

The assembled sheath and trocar are inserted through the stab wound at the chosen point of entry. Although the trocar is reasonably sharp, a moderate amount of force and a rotatory screwing type of motion are needed to penetrate the capsule. The capsule and synovium then form a tight seal around the sheath and minimize leakage of the irrigating fluid. Because this technique necessitates pushing firmly against distended soft tissues, it is important to avoid a sudden plunge which could damage the underlying articular cartilage of the femoral condyles. The scope is therefore held firmly in the palm of the hand with one or two fingers extended (Fig. 3-12). The knee is held in 30°–45° of flexion, and the barrel of the scope is kept parallel to the tibial plateau and directed toward the intercondylar notch.

The trocar is removed and the blunt obturator is inserted before passing the scope into the suprapatellar pouch. This is done by lifting the lower pole of the

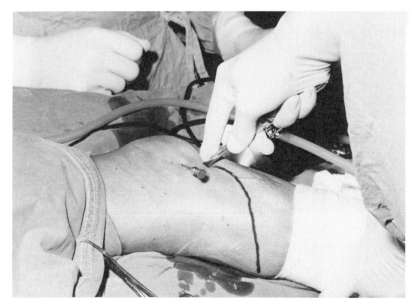

Fig. 3-12.   The sheath and trocar are inserted with the knee flexed 30°; fingers are extended to prevent plunging. The direction of penetration is toward the intercondylar notch.

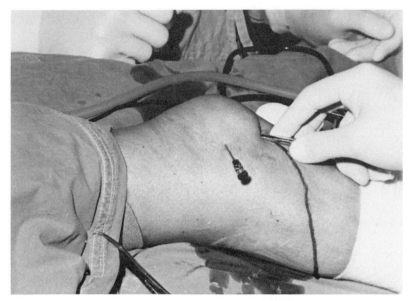

Fig. 3-13.   When the capsule has been broached, the trocar is replaced by the blunt obturator, the knee is extended, and the sheath is passed beneath the patella into the suprapatellar pouch.

patella with the tip of the obturator, straightening the patient's leg, and driving the instrument home between the patella and the underlying femur. The tip then lies in the suprapatellar pouch (Fig. 3-13). With practice, this maneuver can be done quite smoothly and synchronously, without scratching the patellar or femoral articular surfaces.

EXAMINATION OF WASHINGS

When the sheath is in the suprapatellar pouch, the trocar is removed and the washings of the joint are collected and examined for loose bodies or cartilaginous fragments. Synovial fluid cell blocks can be prepared for histological examination of the microscopic joint debris. If the washings contain blood or excessive debris, the joint should be washed clear by opening the stopcock, blocking the exit of the sheath with the thumb, and filling the joint with saline. The thumb is then removed and the washings are examined again. When the outflow is finally clear, the instrument can be fully assembled and the examination begun.

ASSEMBLING THE INSTRUMENT

The instrument is assembled and dismantled when the sheath is in the suprapatellar pouch, where there is sufficient room distal to the tip to perform this operation safely.

After the obturator is removed, the light carrier is fitted inside the sheath and is locked in position. The telescope is then nested within the sheath and light carrier. The electric or fiber light cable and irrigation tubes are then attached, and the instrument is ready for use.

The outflow needle can be fitted to a collecting tube, but we have found that the weight of such a tube tends to block the outflow by tilting the needle and pressing its open end against the synovium. We prefer to catch the outflow in a beaker held by an assistant (Fig. 3-14). If the outflow stops, the assistant can rectify the situation immediately.

NORMAL EXAMINATION

The joint should be examined routinely so that no area is overlooked. We shall describe our routine (borrowed from Watanabe), which we suspect every arthroscopist will modify slightly while developing his own technique. It is a

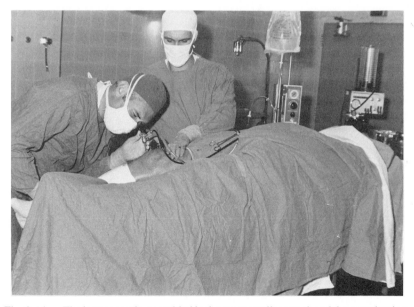

Fig. 3-14.   The instrument is assembled in the suprapatellar pouch and the examination is begun. We prefer to catch the outflow of the irrigating fluid in a beaker held by an assistant. If the outflow becomes blocked, the assistant can rectify the situation quickly.

good policy to scan the whole knee in the routine way, then return to any suspect area for more detailed study.

Suprapatellar Pouch

The table is raised to an appropriate height and the examiner kneels or sits beside the patient (Fig. 3-15). This position allows the examiner to look with the least discomfort directly along the line of the femur into the suprapatellar pouch.

Despite precautions, contamination may occur at this early stage of the examination because the surgeon's cap and mask come very close to and may actually contact the patient's leg. Therefore, we *never touch the barrel* of the arthroscope once the instrument has been inserted.

The tip of the arthroscope is then moved back and forth and the distended suprapatellar pouch is scanned. The sizes of the structures within the joint are determined by gently "pistoning" the arthroscope or moving it in and out so that the changing field gives an idea of perspective and distance. This is also a

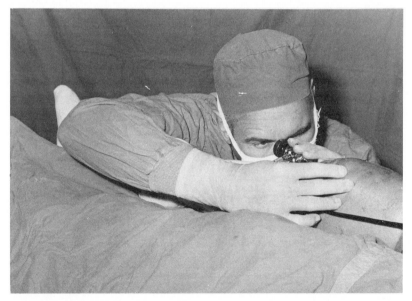

Fig. 3-15.   Examination of the suprapatellar pouch with the knee extended and the arthroscope close to the lower leg. The examiner can tilt and displace the patella from side to side with his free hand for a better view of its articular surface.

good opportunity to make sure that the tip of the outflow irrigation needle is correctly placed and is not likely to be blocked by synovial fronds, debris, or adhesions.

The size, shape, and color of the synovial fronds in the area must be closely examined. Check carefully for hypertrophy of synovium in the parapatellar region (parapatellar fringe).

The plica suprapatellaris is seen as a crescentic fold on the medial side of the suprapatellar pouch (Fig. 3-16, see Plate 1) and may extend across the pouch to divide it almost in two. Sometimes it is so pronounced that only a narrow porta leads into the quadriceps bursa. The plica suprapatellaris is not usually of any pathological significance, and its size is variable. Occasionally, the plica is markedly thickened and bandlike, and then it may be considered pathological.

Patellofemoral Joint

As the arthroscope is withdrawn from the suprapatellar pouch, a crescent of light appears in the upper part of the field. This is the undersurface of the patella, seen tangentially or in profile much like the radiographic "skyline" view (Fig. 3-16). At this point, the tip of the scope is just beneath the inferior pole of the patella. Using his free hand, the surgeon palpates the upper pole of the patella and tilts it slightly to better visualize the undersurface. Also, the medial and lateral facets can be seen by sweeping the scope from side to side or by medial or lateral displacement of the patella using the free hand.

The tip of the outflow needle may also be used as a probe to identify areas of articular cartilage softening on the patella.

If the Watanabe 21 is being used, it must be lying flat at this point, rather than vertical. That is to say, the instrument should be turned so that the narrowest diameter of the lens and light combination is passed through this area. The relative positions of the light and lens can always be determined by the position of the proximal electric post, as the post is on the same side as the distal light.

If a fore-oblique instrument is used (e.g., Storz), it should be rotated through 180° with the lens facing upwards to inspect the undersurface of the patella.

As the arthroscope is withdrawn gently from the patellofemoral compartment, the congruence of the femoral notch and the patellar surface can be determined, but bear in mind that the tip of the scope may lift the lower pole of the patella and cause a slight change in the contact areas.

When the patellofemoral compartment has been cleared, the tip of the scope suddenly becomes free, and the medial compartment can be entered.

Medial Compartment

The medial compartment is entered with a smooth and synchronous movement of head, hand, and body that requires some practice. The patient's heel is lowered over the edge of the table to flex the knee, while the tip of the arthroscope is allowed to orbit the perimeter of the femoral condyle (Fig. 3-17). This can be done by keeping the horizon of the femoral condyle in view as the knee is slowly flexed. The eyepiece of the scope rises as the tip of the scope descends into the anterior part of the medial compartment and the anterior horn of the medial meniscus comes into view (Fig. 3-16).

With the Watanabe 21, it is best to perform this movement with the light carrier leading the lens, and supported by the telescope following behind. Adhesions, plicae, or bands in the medial gutter can catch on the slightly protruding bulb and bend it outward if it is not supported by the telescope during this movement.

With the knee flexed 30°–40°, the tip of the scope should be lying on the anterior horn of the medial meniscus. The meniscosynovial junction is easily

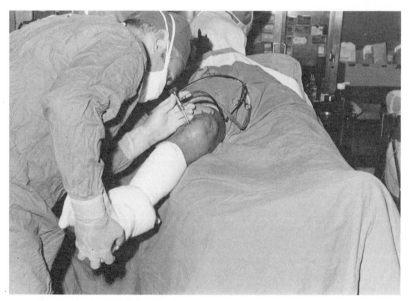

Fig. 3-17. The medial compartment is examined with the knee flexed by dropping the foot over the side of the table and applying a mild valgus strain.

identified by the transition from pink synovium to white meniscus (if the tourniquet has not been inflated). The next landmark is the free inner border of the meniscus. When the smooth, knifelike edge of the meniscus is seen clearly, it is followed posteriorly with the knee in slight flexion and neutral rotation. The inner border of the meniscus can be followed to the posteromedial area where the arc of the femoral condyle usually obscures vision. The posterior horn may then be seen lateral to the condyle (Fig. 3-16). For the best view, an assistant steadies the lower end of the femur while the examiner applies a strong valgus strain to the knee by abducting the heel with his other hand. The joint opens maximally at 20°–30° of flexion. If this is still not sufficient to permit a satisfactory view of the posterior horn, the instrument can be used for gentle prying. Direct pressure with the scope tends to spread the femoral condyle away from the tibial plateau and permit an even better view of the posterior horn and the posteromedial corner of the joint. However, often a "blind spot" persists in this area, and the integrity of the meniscus must be assessed by closely examining the contour of the inner border of the meniscus and by looking for telltale signs of articular cartilage degeneration on the femoral condyle. A small "flounce" is often seen on the inner border of the meniscus when the tibia is rotated. This is normal and must not be confused with a pathological condition (Fig. 3-16). Identification of meniscal lesions is discussed in detail in Chapter 5.

After examining the posterior horn, the surgeon returns the arthroscope to the front of the joint in order to examine the articular cartilage of the femoral condyle. With the scope held against the top of the anterior horn of the medial meniscus, the knee is slowly flexed from 0° to beyond a right angle. During this procedure, the scope rides with the tibia and sweeps across the weight-bearing surface of the medial femoral condyle. The normal condyle is smooth and white. Areas of chondromalacia can be identified by patches of fibrillated cartilage or by actual areas of erosion, the edges of which cast shadows that change with the movement of the light. Articular cartilage diseases will also be discussed more fully in Chapter 5.

The next maneuver is to apply rotational stress while watching the inner border of the meniscus. Occasionally, the meniscus moves in or out of its natural position, indicating a possible disruption of its peripheral attachments.

A second hypodermic needle, usually 18 gauge, can be inserted at the joint line to improve irrigation and to act as a probe for detecting areas of articular cartilage damage or identifying peripheral detachments or lacerations in the main body of the meniscus (Fig. 5-2).

The tibial plateau is finally examined before leaving the medial compartment. This plateau is usually featureless except for the occasional evidence of chondromalacia.

Intercondylar Notch

The tip of the scope is now moved toward the intercondylar region where the scope is placed on the anterior cruciate ligament. The anterior cruciate is covered with synovium, and a longitudinally oriented vascular pattern can often be seen. The insertion of the anterior cruciate is magnified by its proximity to the lens, and the ligament appears to taper upward toward its origin in the intercondylar notch (Fig. 3-16). Anteriorly on the lateral border of the medial femoral condyle, a small synovial-covered mound is frequently seen, which represents the origin of the posterior cruciate ligament. Normally, the rest of the posterior cruciate cannot be seen because the anterior cruciate obscures it. The alar or suspensory ligament is occasionally seen and may sometimes be perforated by the trocar at the time of insertion. If this happens, it may be difficult to move the tip of the scope from the intercondylar region to the lateral compartment.

Lateral Compartment

With the tip of the scope in the center of the knee and lying on top of the anterior cruciate, it is safe to lift the leg onto the table and flex the knee to approximately 80°. When the lateral border of the heel is supported on the operating table, the whole leg tends to fall into external rotation at the hip. A varus strain can then be applied to the knee by gentle downward pressure on the medial aspect of the joint (Fig. 3-18). This opens the lateral compartment widely, and it is usually simple to slip the tip of the arthroscope sideways into the compartment. If this maneuver is difficult, it is usually because the arthroscope is caught on the alar suspensory ligament, or else an intercondylar septum is present. If the intercondylar notch cannot be traversed easily, it is prudent to remove the scope and reinsert it from an anteromedial approach.

In the lateral compartment, the posterior horn of the lateral meniscus is the first structure seen. With the knee in flexion and after a varus strain is applied, the posterior region opens quite widely. Visualization is aided by the slightly convex surface of the tibial plateau. The posterior horn of the lateral meniscus normally dips down behind the posterior edge of the tibia, where it is securely anchored, and its attachments to the ligaments of Humphrey and Wrisberg cannot normally be identified. However, if a fore-oblique lens is used, these ligaments and the posterior cruciate may sometimes be seen.

The inner border of the meniscus is identified near its posterior attachment, and the contour of the inner border is assessed by following it to the front of the joint. The popliteus tendon can sometimes be seen as it courses obliquely

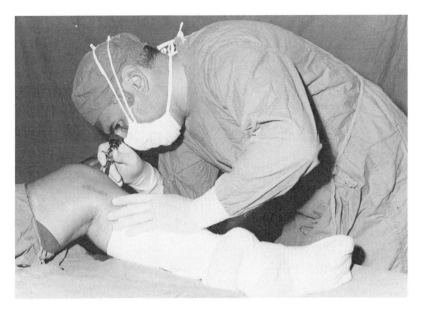

Fig. 3-18. The lateral compartment is examined by placing the heel on the table and applying gentle varus strain by pressing downward on the flexed knee.

through the posterolateral corner of the joint (Fig. 3-16). The space through which it runs should not be confused with a peripheral tear of the meniscus. The anterior horn of the lateral meniscus is difficult to assess from the usual anterolateral approach because of its proximity to the lens. (If the surgeon is concerned about disease in this area, an anteromedial approach is advised.)

The lateral meniscus is broader than the medial and can spread halfway across the articular surface. Discoid menisci are often missed because they completely cover the tibial plateau, and their inner edge, which is adjacent to the intercondylar notch, is not appreciated. The tight C-shaped border of the meniscus must always be identified and followed from back to front because it is the key to determining the integrity of the meniscus.

Before ending the examination of the lateral compartment, the surgeon also scans the articular cartilage of the femoral condyle by holding the arthroscope steady and moving the tibia as already described.

If loose bodies are suspected, the lateral gutter can be examined by moving the arthroscope from the suprapatellar pouch, over the lateral femoral condyle, and directly down the lateral recess. Palpation or ballottement with the free hand sometimes floats a "loose body" into view.

SECOND INSERTIONS

Should a second insertion be needed, it is wise to inflate the tourniquet before withdrawing the instrument from the first point of entry. If this is not done, bleeding from the original entry wound may quickly obscure the field of vision and unnecessarily delay the examination. After the tourniquet is inflated, the first point of entry is sutured, the joint is again distended by injecting normal saline through the outflow needle, and the second insertion is made from the other side of the joint.

BIOPSIES

Biopsies can be obtained in two ways. In the first, an area is selected (usually in the suprapatellar pouch or the medial compartment), the telescope is removed, the biopsy forceps is inserted, and the area is sampled blindly. This type of biopsy usually yields enough tissue for diagnosis, but if a specific lesion is the target (e.g., crystal synovitis or synovial chondromatosis), the second type of biopsy—biopsy under direct vision (Fig. 3-19)—is recommended. A second sheath, through which the biopsy forceps is manipulated, is inserted into the joint. With some arthroscopes, biopsy under direct vision is facilitated by inserting a narrower telescope down the original sheath, thus also providing space for the biopsy forceps.

PHOTOGRAPHY

Most manufacturers supply a modified single-lens reflex camera that can be attached to the eyepiece of their particular arthroscope. An unsterile assistant can attach the camera to the scope and take the picture, while the sterile examiner steadies the scope, looks through the viewfinder, and selects his field (Fig. 3-20). In most instruments, the light for photography is not great, and the exposure may of necessity be relatively long. The assistant must therefore hold the camera very still during exposure, particularly if the selected shutter speed is less than 1/30 second. When the shutter release button is pressed, a second light circuit or flash generator momentarily increases the light intensity to the correct level.

Although the camera can be sterilized with gas so that the examiner can hold it himself, film which is gas sterilized more than four times reportedly

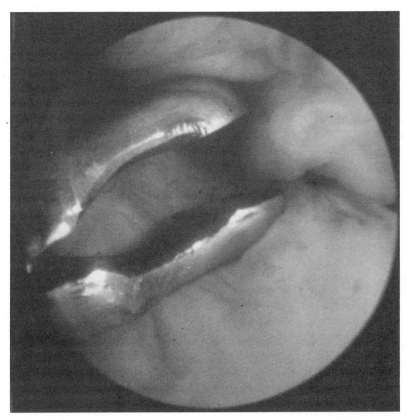

Fig. 3-19.   Biopsy under direct vision is possible when the biopsy forceps is introduced through a second sheath.

tends to lose its emulsion. High-speed Ektachrome Type B (adjusted for artificial light) is used with the Watanabe 21 arthroscope. High-speed daylight type films should be used with fiber light arthroscopes. As the shutter speed and aperture size vary from instrument to instrument, the manufacturers' instructions should be followed and some trial exposures carried out.

A method must also be established for relating the patient to the photograph. One solution is to use a single roll of film for each case, but this can be expensive and wasteful. We record as many cases as possible on each roll of film, separating each case with two blank frames. The film is developed but not mounted. The photographs are then related to the correct patient by referring to the order of the examinations. Leaving the film unmounted makes storage (for

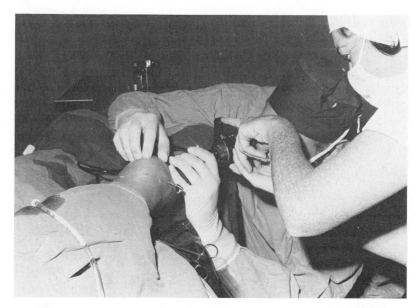

Fig. 3-20.   A single-lens reflex camera is held by an unsterile assistant.

record purposes) easier and the accumulation of mounted slides (for teaching purposes) more selective.

A final practical recommendation for photography is to take the pictures so that they are easily oriented when they are later projected or otherwise studied. No matter what position the leg is in when the photograph is taken, the tibial plateaus will always be in the bottom of the final picture if the camera body is oriented at right angles to the long axis of the tibia when the shutter is released.

CONCLUDING THE EXAMINATION

Concluding the examination involves a retracing of steps. The scope is brought back to the intercondylar region, and the anterior cruciate, and adjacent structures are reexamined before moving back into the medial compartment for a final look at any suspicious areas. The foot is again lowered over the edge of the table, and the scope is brought back around the medial femoral condyle into the patellofemoral pouch as the knee is straightened. This is the end of the examination. The tourniquet is released (if it had been inflated), the telescope is withdrawn, and the light carrier is removed. But before the sheath is removed, the joint is irrigated constantly until all bleeding has subsided and the washings are clear. The sheath is then slowly withdrawn, the irrigating outflow needles are removed, and the suprapatellar pouch is compressed to squeeze excess fluid out as the sheath is removed. The wound is closed with a single deep stitch embracing as much subcutaneous tissue as possible. A small dressing is applied over the suture, and an elasticized bandage is wrapped around the knee. The patient can walk immediately after awakening from the anesthetic. The suture is usually removed 7 days later. Showers are permitted at any time, but the patients are advised not to soak in a bathtub until at least 48 hours have elapsed following removal of the suture.

ARTHROTOMY FOLLOWING ARTHROSCOPY

If a surgically treatable lesion is detected at arthroscopy and the patient is under general anesthesia, arthrotomy can be performed under the same anesthetic. However, we recommend arthrotomy as a separate procedure. We therefore withdraw the scope, close the arthroscopy wound with a single stitch, cover the area with a sterile towel, and remove all drapes that were used for the arthroscopic examination. The tourniquet can then be inflated after exsanguination of the leg with an Esmarch bandage. The skin is prepared again, and the operating team changes gowns and gloves. New drapes are applied, and the arthrotomy is done as if it were a fresh case.

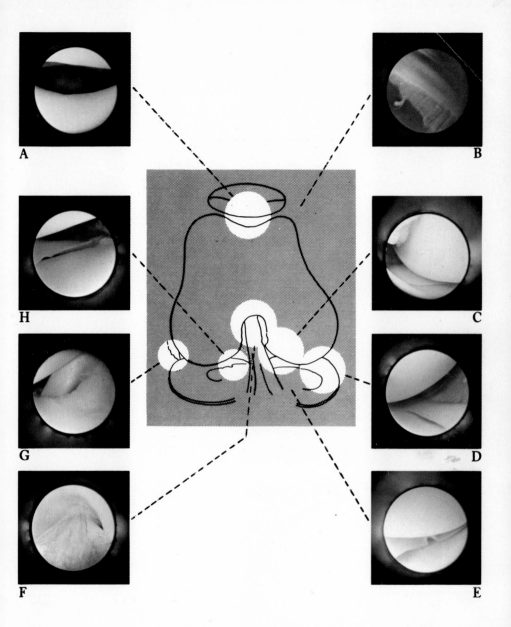

Fig. 3-16. Typical views of a normal knee. (B.) Plica suprapatellaris (A.) tangential view of patellofemoral articulation (C.) posterior horn, medial meniscus (D.) anterior region, medial meniscus (F.) anterior cruciate (G.) popliteus tendon (H.) posterior horn, lateral meniscus (E.) normal "flounce," medial meniscus.

Plate 1

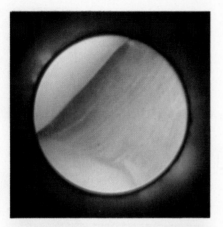

Fig. 4-1. Synovium, medial compartment, in a 22-year-old patient with a normal knee.

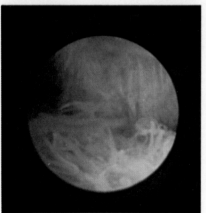

Fig. 4-2. Synovium, suprapatellar pouch, in a 50-year-old patient with a normal knee.

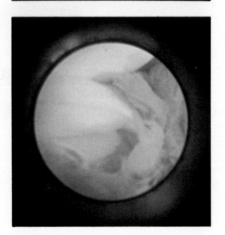

Fig. 4-3. Post-traumatic synovitis 6 months after bucket-handle tear of medial meniscus.

Plate 2

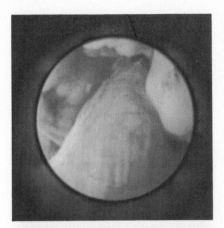

Fig. 4-4. Degenerative arthritis in a 55-year-old patient. Synovium overlying anterior cruciate is hyperemic, and fronds at upper left are hypertrophied. Osteophyte present at upper right; fibrin strands, lower left.

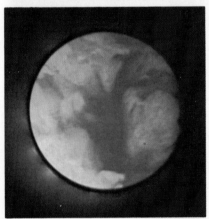

Fig. 4-5. Rheumatoid arthritis, early acute stage. Note club-shaped hypertrophy of synovial fronds and irregular hyperemia.

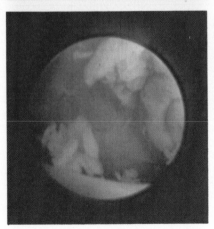

Fig. 4-6. Rheumatoid arthritis—late stage. Note pannus *(upper right),* necrotic synovial fronds (white), fibrinous rice bodies *(lower left),* and abnormal articular cartilage in central background.

Plate 3

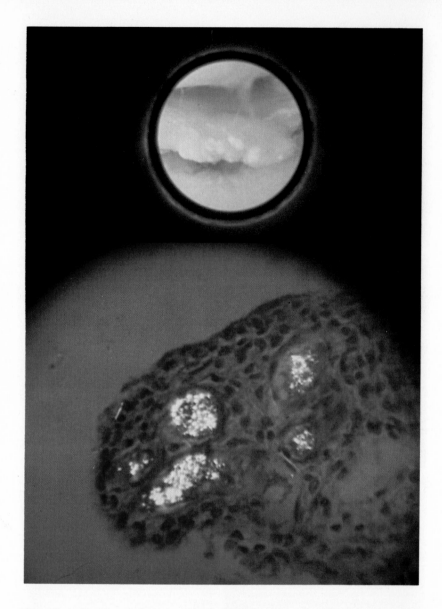

Fig. 4-7. Crystal synovitis (chondrocalcinosis). Crystal deposits noted in degenerative meniscal tissue *(top)*. Synovial biopsy examined under polarized light *(bottom)* shows birefringent crystals of calcium pyrophosphate. (Courtesy Dr. R. O'Connor.)

Plate 4

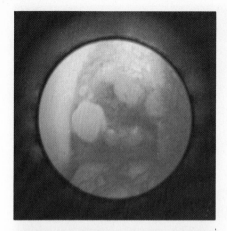

Fig. 4-8. Synovial osteochondromatosis. Metaplastic changes in synovium produce calcified loose bodies.

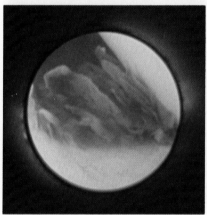

Fig. 4-9. Pigmented villonodular synovitis. Note shaggy, brown, hyperemic, and hypertrophied synovium.

Plate 5

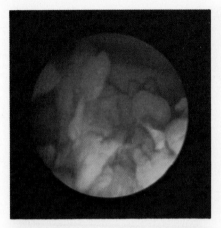

Fig. 4-10. Hemophilic arthritis. Hypertrophied synovium resembles that seen in chronic inflammation (due to repeated hemarthrosis).

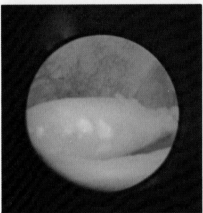

Fig. 4-11. Xanthoma ($20 \times 8 \times 5$ mm) arising from synovium in suprapatellar pouch.

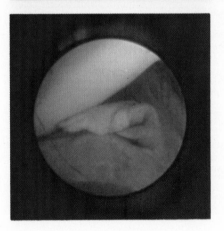

Fig. 4-12. Pinched synovial fronds —anteromedial compartment.

Plate 6

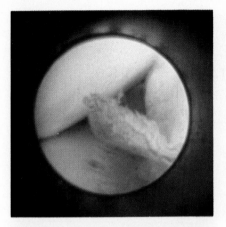

Fig. 4-13. Pinched synovial frond
—anteromedial compartment.

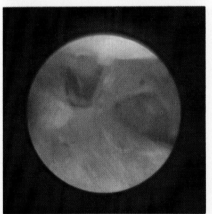

Fig. 4-14. Adhesions (early)—supra-patellar pouch, post-traumatic.

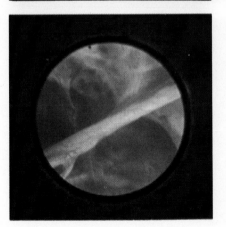

Fig. 4-15. Adhesions (mature)—su-prapatellar pouch, post-traumatic.

Plate 7

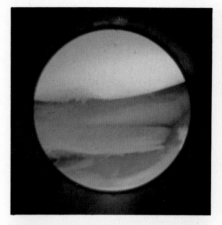

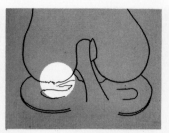

Fig. 4-16. Longitudinal tear, posterior horn of lateral meniscus. Note small area of condylar chondromalacia.

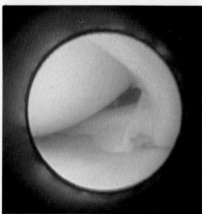

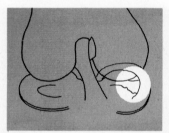

Fig. 4-19. Anterior horn region and peripheral rim of bucket-handle tear. Displaced portion rises above the tip of the arthroscope.

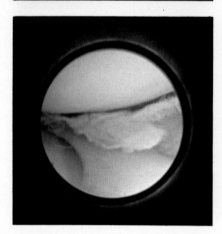

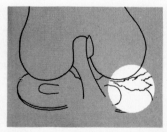

Fig. 4-25. Fresh posterior horn flap tear of medial meniscus.

Plate 8

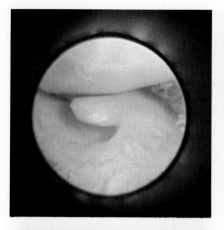

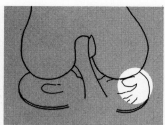

Fig. 4-26. Chronic posterior horn flap tear of medial meniscus. Edges of flap are smooth due to attrition.

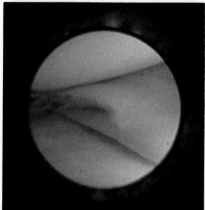

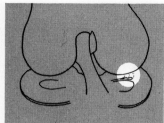

Fig. 4-30. Horizontal cleavage tear of posterior horn, medial meniscus, with inward displacement of the superior fragment.

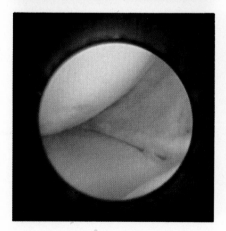

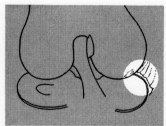

Fig. 4-34. Medial compartment 1 year after meniscectomy. Note early degenerative changes on femoral condyle and minimal regeneration of meniscus.

Plate 9

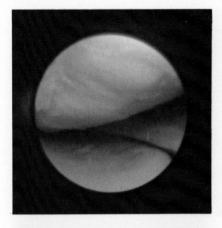

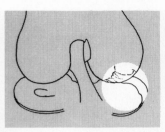

Fig. 4-35. Medial compartment 30 years after meniscectomy. Degenerative changes on articular cartilage are more marked, and meniscal regeneration is minimal.

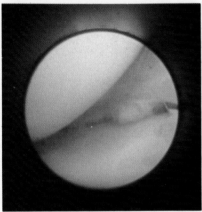

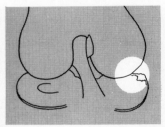

Fig. 4-36. Small tear in peripheral rim after medial meniscectomy.

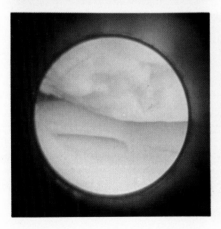

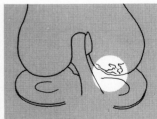

Fig. 4-40. Donor site on medial femoral condyle of cartilaginous loose body found in suprapatellar pouch.

Plate 10

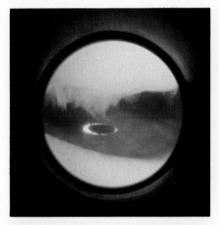

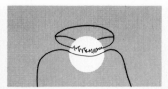

Fig. 4-44. Grade I chondromalacia patellae—localized fibrillation of patella with no changes on femoral surface.

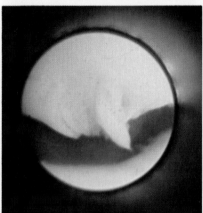

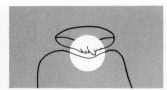

Fig. 4-45. Grade II chondromalacia patellae—extensive fibrillation or fragmentation of the patella with a normal femoral surface.

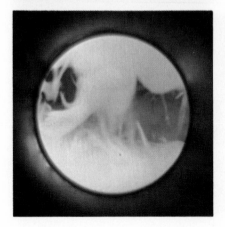

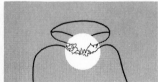

Fig. 4-46. Grade III chondromalacia patellae—degenerative changes on both sides of the patellofemoral articulation.

Plate 11

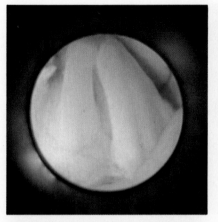

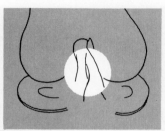

Fig. 4-49. Normal intact and bifurcated anterior cruciate ligament.

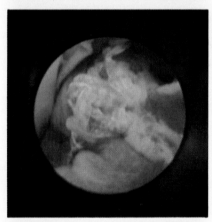

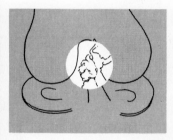

Fig. 4-50. Complete recent rupture of midportion of anterior cruciate.

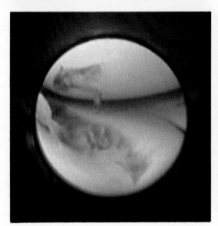

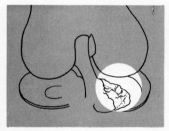

Fig. 4-51. Distal avulsion of anterior cruciate with fragment of bone attached.

Plate 12

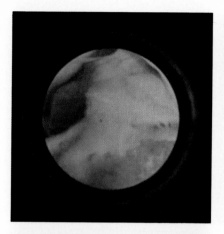

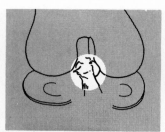

Fig. 4-52. Partial rupture of anterior cruciate with intact synovial sheath and subsynovial hemorrhages.

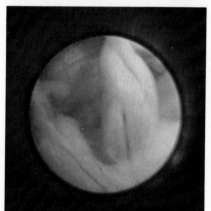

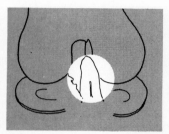

Fig. 4-53. Old tear of anterior cruciate with rounding off of the distal stub of ligament.

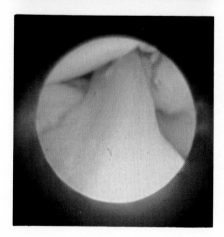

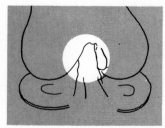

Fig. 4-54. Normal anterior cruciate with the origin of posterior cruciate covered by a small fat pad visible on the lateral border of the medial femoral condyle *(top right)*.

Plate 13

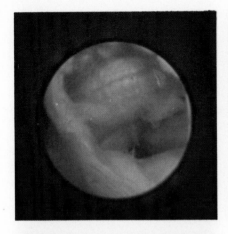

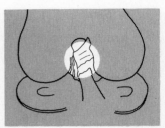

Fig. 4-55. Posterior cruciate ligament is usually seen only when the anterior cruciate is torn.

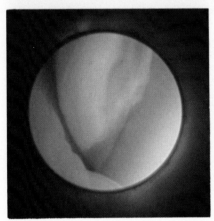

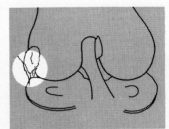

Fig. 4-56. Avulsion of the popliteus tendon insertion. Avulsed fragment of bone *(center)* is pulled into an intra-articular site by popliteus tendon, seen at distal tip.

Plate 14

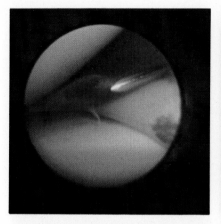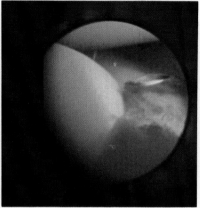

Fig. 5-2. Hypodermic needle (18 gauge) inserted at joint line improves irrigation and can also be used as a probe.

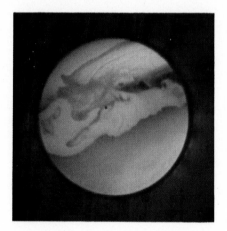

Fig. 5-4. Large mass of fibrin that was misdiagnosed as a torn meniscus; false-positive error.

Plate 15

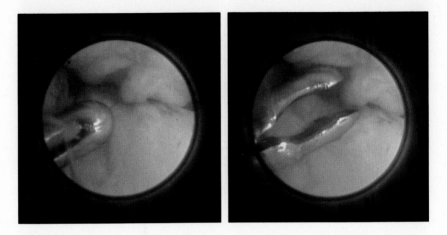

Fig. 6-2.   Biopsy of synovium under direct vision. Biopsy forceps is introduced through a separate sheath.

Plate 16

4
Pathological Conditions

This chapter is not intended as an atlas of joint pathology. It is intended as a guide to the recognition of some of the pathological conditions that can occur within a knee joint. It is therefore presented in a way that we feel is practical for the arthroscopist.

Although not knowing fully what to expect, the arthroscopist usually suspects abnormalities in the synovial lining, the menisci, the patellar or condylar articular cartilage, or the ligamentous structures. Consequently, he tends to concentrate on each of these in turn. Once fully informed about the type and extent of pathological findings within the joint, he can better decide future management.

SYNOVIAL DISORDERS

Although normal synovium in a young knee is smooth, red to reddish pink, and generally unimpressive (Fig. 4-1, see Plate 2), it becomes increasingly hypertrophied with age, and one must be careful not to interpret the fine but normal synovial tufting in the suprapatellar area of a 50-year-old patient's knee as pathological (Fig. 4-2, see Plate 2). Also, the type of synovial proliferation may be diagnostic for certain diseases, but we are inclined to believe that synovial response is generally nonspecific and that its appearance depends largely on the severity and duration of the inflammatory stimulus.

45

Acute Inflammation

Synovial alterations due to post-traumatic or reactive synovitis do not resemble those of old age. There are varying degrees of edema, hypertrophy, and hyperemia (Fig. 4-3, see Plate 2). A full-blown inflammatory response of this kind takes 2 or 3 days to develop and may be caused by many things in addition to direct or indirect trauma. A similar reaction is produced by desquamated fragments of articular cartilage in chondromalacia, after infection, entrapment of synovial fronds, hemarthrosis, and the injection of radioopaque agents used for arthrography. As the fibrin content of the synovial effusion is increased, mucinous strands of fibrin may also be seen.

Osteoarthritis

In osteoarthritis, the changes resemble those seen in acute inflammation but are accentuated possibly because of chronic irritation due to microfragments of articular cartilage debris. The synovial fronds in osteoarthritis are typically filiform (Fig. 4-4, see Plate 3) and usually different from those of acute inflammation or rheumatoid arthritis. (The articular cartilage changes in osteoarthritis are described later.)

Rheumatoid Arthritis

In rheumatoid arthritis and such allied systemic disorders as psoriatic arthritis, the synovium exhibits a characteristic clublike proliferation. The fronds are thick, bulbous, and bright red because of an intense hyperemia (Fig. 4-5, see Plate 3). Areas of fibrin deposition appear brilliant white against the deeper crimson of the inflamed synovium (Fig. 4-6, see Plate 3). The tips of the rheumatoid fronds may become necrotic and also appear white because of loss of blood supply. It is postulated that these necrotic tips of synovium sometimes break away, become enveloped in a layer of fibrin, and form the "rice bodies" frequently seen in cases of far-advanced rheumatoid arthritis.

Crystal Synovitis

At first glance, crystal synovitis appears as a nonspecific inflammatory response with hyperemia and moderate hypertrophy, but on closer examination small refractile crystalline bodies can be seen sparkling in the light. The crystals may be densely studded throughout the joint, or they may be sparse and require careful searching before discovery. Occasionally, whole fronds are encrusted with crystals and glitter like a small Christmas tree. Biopsies have shown that these crystals are usually calcium pyrophosphate and occasionally uric acid (Fig. 4-7, see Plate 4).

Osteochondromatosis

In the early stages of osteochondromatosis, small white but nonrefractile cartilaginous bodies stud or seed the inflamed synovium (Fig. 4-8, see Plate 5). In the later stages, these bodies are stalked and may detach to become loose bodies.

Pigmented Villonodular Synovitis

Pigmented villonodular synovitis has a characteristic appearance as a result of recurrent hemarthrosis. The synovium is stained brown, and it is shaggy, proliferative, and fairly uniform in appearance (Fig. 4-9, see Plate 5).

Hemophilic Arthritis

Hemophilic arthritis resembles pigmented villonodular synovitis except that in our experience, in the former the fronds tend to be plumper and more suggestive of an acute reaction than a chronic state (Fig. 4-10, see Plate 6).

Xanthoma

On one occasion we saw a xanthoma (Fig. 4-11, see Plate 6) arising in the suprapatellar pouch. The tumor was stalked and was associated with recurrent synovial effusions.

Trapped Synovium

In 1904 Hoffa described a syndrome affecting the fat pad at the front of the joint. His description was based on clinical observation and gross physical findings. We believe there is a spectrum of conditions ranging from Hoffa's classical syndrome to early post-traumatic hypertrophy of a single pinched synovial frond (Fig. 4-12, see Plate 6). Many large synovial fronds may be nipped between the articular surfaces, or a single frond can become so swollen and engorged that it resembles a strangulated hemorrhoid (Fig. 4-13, see Plate 7). A fall on the knee or a twisting strain due to playing football might pinch a synovial frond, which then swells and becomes increasingly vulnerable to repeated entrapment between the articular surfaces as the knee comes into full extension. If the swelling and pinching persist, the condition may progress to the classical Hoffa's syndrome.

Adhesions

Adhesions may be seen after trauma, surgery, or acute inflammation and in many instances seem to be responsible for vague, aching discomfort in the knee. These are quite different from the gross adhesions that limit the range of motion of the joint after severe trauma. Occasionally, as one distends the joint before inserting the arthroscope the adhesions (Fig. 4-14, see Plate 7), pop in a fine crepitant or crackling fashion.

In some instances, thick bands of fibrous tissue are seen, usually with blood vessels crossing from one synovial surface to another (Fig. 4-15, see Plate 7). In other instances, sheets of filmy adhesions can be broken by moving the scope or the irrigating needle around in the suprapatellar pouch. Rupture of these adhesions often relieves vague symptoms.

MENISCAL PATHOLOGY

Lacerations

Longitudinal (Fig. 4-16, see Plate 8) or transverse (Fig. 4-20) lacerations are by far the most common meniscal lesions and may be seen in any part of either meniscus. Most lacerations can be detected easily during the routine examination described in Chapter 3.

A bucket-handle tear with the displaced portion lying in the intercondylar notch can create difficulties for the novice (Fig. 4-17). The displaced fragment may prevent the scope from entering the opposite compartment and obscure vision completely. However, this in itself is diagnostic of the abnormality. With care, one can usually bypass this mass and visualize the anterior horn well

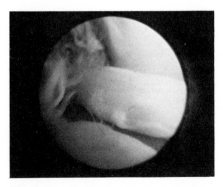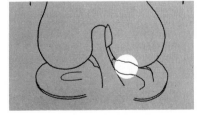

Fig. 4-17.   Bucket-handle tear of medial meniscus with displaced portion lying in the intercondylar notch and blocking the view of the peripheral rim.

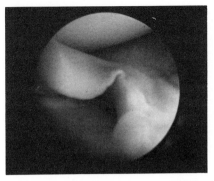
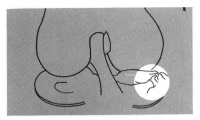

Fig. 4-18.   Anterior horn region of bucket-handle tear, with displaced portion rising to the left to enter the intercondylar notch.

enough to see that it is the meniscus folded upon itself (Fig. 4-18). Sometimes the posterior horn attachment can also be seen. If the fragment is fairly loose or detached posteriorly, the scope can often be slipped above or beneath the fragment to reveal the peripheral rim, which is then inspected for additional tears (Fig. 4-19, see Plate 8). Occasionally, a meniscus may be split along its length but remain undisplaced. If so, the meniscus lies in its usual position and its inner border appears normal. The split can be revealed by inserting a second needle at the joint line and using it to displace the meniscus toward the intercondylar notch and to open the cleft in its substance.

Transverse lacerations of the meniscus are more common on the lateral side than on the medial (Fig. 4-20). They usually result from an inward displacement of the meniscus with the anterior and posterior horns still tethered. Therefore, the inner border is stretched, and the meniscus splits

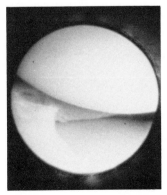
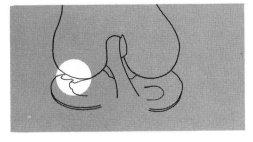

Fig. 4-20.   Transverse laceration of lateral meniscus.

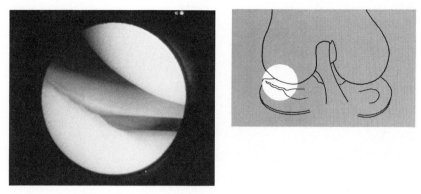

Fig. 4-21.   Transverse laceration of lateral meniscus.

transversely (Fig. 4-21). The use of the probing needle is helpful in delineating this abnormality.

Peripheral Separations

A peripheral separation in the posteromedial corner of the meniscus can be particularly difficult to demonstrate, but it should be suspected if the inner border of the meniscus slides toward the center of the joint on external rotation in slight valgus (Fig. 4-22). However, this inward bulging, incurving, or pouting of the inner border (Fig. 4-23) must be interpreted in the light of other findings, such as articular cartilage changes in the area. It might also be considered a positive finding if the patient's history is strongly suggestive of an unstable meniscus or if there is abnormal laxity of the medial ligament or

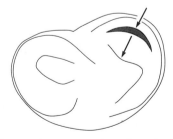

Fig. 4-22.   A peripheral separation or tear of meniscus in the posteromedial corner allows the meniscus to bulge inward toward the center of the joint. This is seen as a change in the contour of the inner border of the meniscus.

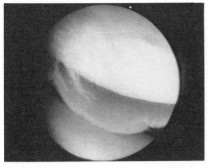 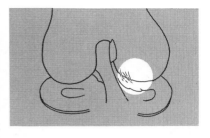

Fig. 4-23.   Inbulging of posterior horn of medial meniscus is strongly suggestive of a tear or peripheral separation. Degenerative changes in the articular cartilage provide additional evidence of a posteromedial tear.

capsule (Fig. 4-24). The probing needle may be extremely helpful in demonstrating these lesions.

If after adequate examination the integrity of the posterior horn of the medial meniscus is still in doubt, arthrography may be helpful. However, the posterior horn of the lateral meniscus is seen far better at arthroscopy than at arthrography because the lateral compartment opens widely, usually revealing the entire superior surface of the meniscus.

Flaps and Tags

Meniscal flaps or tags (Fig. 4-25, 4-26, see Plates 8 and 9, and Fig. 4-27) result from small splits along the inner border of the meniscus and are most common toward the anterior horn. They are not usually large enough to cause

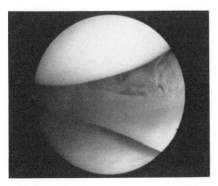 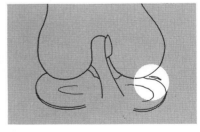

Fig. 4-24.   Abnormal laxity of medial collateral ligament after trauma permits easy examination of the meniscus. The meniscus is intact, but a small split in the synovium is seen at the meniscosynovial junction.

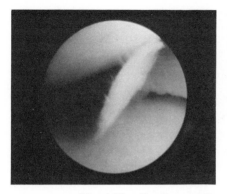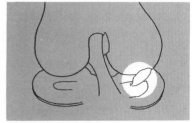

Fig. 4-27.   Small recent flap tear of medial meniscus.

episodes of true locking, but they cause a sensation of instability as they move
in and out of the weight-bearing area between the femoral condyle and the tibial
plateau. We feel that if these flaps or tags are small, all that is needed to abolish
the sensation of instability is a partial meniscectomy to remove the offending
portion. This procedure can often be performed through the arthroscope with
grasping forceps (Fig. 4-28). Large lacerations of the anterior horn are exceed-
ingly rare.

Cleavage Tears

Horizontal cleavage tears, usually seen in the posterior horn, result from
degenerative changes that allow horizontal splits to develop from the shear
stresses applied to the posterior horns (Fig. 4-29). During flexion, the upper
surface of the meniscus slides over the inferior surface; the inner border bulges
suspiciously inward, changing the normally congruous curve of the inner

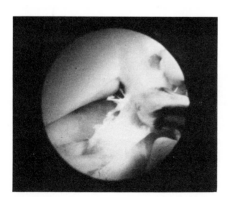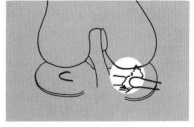

Fig. 4-28.   Grasping forceps are used to remove an anterior horn flap tear of a medial
meniscus, i.e., a partial meniscectomy is done with the aid of the arthroscope.

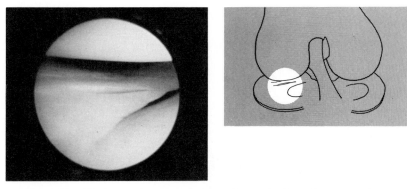

Fig. 4-29. Horizontal "cleavage" tears of posterior horn, lateral meniscus.

border (Fig. 4-30, see Plate 9). Suspicious lesions may be confirmed by lifting the meniscus with a needle and looking for a fissure on the inferior surface. Cleavage lesions cause an aching discomfort in the knee, which is aggravated by activity—particularly bending, stooping, or twisting. The knee does not usually give way or swell, and there is seldom a clear history of precipitating trauma. More lacerations occur in time until the meniscus loses its normal sharp, razorlike edge and becomes a mass of soft tissue through trituration (Fig. 4-31). The articular cartilage adjacent to such a degenerating lesion is usually involved in a degenerative process itself. The prognosis is poor, but most physicians agree that it is better to remove these degenerative menisci as early as possible to minimize the progression of the degenerative changes in the femoral condyle. One wonders, however, whether the loss of the meniscus, even though it is abnormal, might not enhance the degenerative process in the articular cartilage.

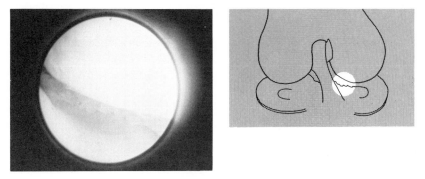

Fig. 4-31. Maceration of posterior horn of medial meniscus.

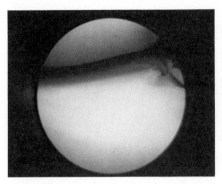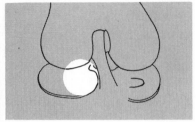

Fig. 4-32. Discoid lateral meniscus. Note inner border of meniscus close to the intercondylar notch.

Discoid Menisci

Discoid menisci are more common on the lateral side but also occur in the medial compartment. The condition can be diagnosed only by finding the inner border of the meniscus near the center of the joint by following its upper surface from the periphery. If a discoid lateral meniscus is suspected, the attachments of the posterior horn should be examined because the meniscus may be loosely inserted into the ligament of Wrisberg rather than firmly attached to the tibia. Discoid menisci (Fig. 4-32) are mobile and bear all the load of the femoral condyle. They are quite vulnerable to traumatic laceration.

Dislocating Menisci

It is sometimes said that "hypermobile meniscus" is a diagnosis of the destitute. Nevertheless, the anterior horns of some medial menisci undoubtedly do dislocate anteriorly as the knee extends, thus allowing the articular cartilage of the tibia and femur to come into direct contact (Fig. 4-33). We do not advocate the routine removal of such menisci, and we cannot state categorically that the condition is pathological. However, dislocating menisci may exist without an associated posterior horn lesion or any other abnormality. Most patients suffer pain on hyperextension, probably due to tibiofemoral impingement. Sometimes their symptoms subside with a short course of anti-inflammatory drugs.

Peripheral Rims and Retained Fragments

Although several cases of significant meniscal reformation after meniscectomy are described in the literature, arthroscopic evidence suggests that this

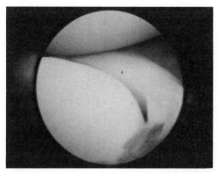 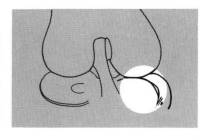

Fig. 4-33.   Dislocating anterior horn of medial meniscus, which can develop after traumatic rupture of the anterior coronary ligament.

is the exception rather than the rule (Fig. 4-34, see Plate 9). Even 30 years after meniscectomy, the peripheral rim is usually no wider than 2–3 mm and is usually composed of soft fibrous tissue rather than resilient fibrocartilage (Fig. 4-35, see Plate 10). If a significant rim is left at the time of meniscectomy, such as after removal of only the displaced portion of a bucket-handle lesion, the inner border soon becomes smoother and, once again, wedge shaped. Additional tears may occur with additional trauma to these reformed or residual rims (Fig. 4-36, see Plate 10), and if no other lesion is found to explain the symptoms, a "rimectomy" may be advisable.

Posterior horn fragments are frequently left at the time of surgery, particularly if a small anterior incision is used (Fig. 4-37). Surprisingly, however, these fragments are not the most common cause of trouble after meniscectomy. But if a retained fragment is large, it may interfere with the normal synchronous movement of the joint by creating an unbalanced compartment and thereby promote degenerative changes on the femoral condyles. We do not advocate removing every retained posterior horn that is detected, but we advise removing the larger fragments, particularly if there is any condylar chondromalacia.

ARTICULAR CARTILAGE

Lesions of the articular cartilage have long been neglected. At arthrotomy, gross lesions can easily be identified, but lesser abnormalities are seldom noticed. When one examines the knee through a magnifying lens and in the presence of a fast-flowing stream of saline, the differences between normal and abnormal cartilage are quite obvious.

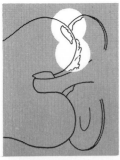

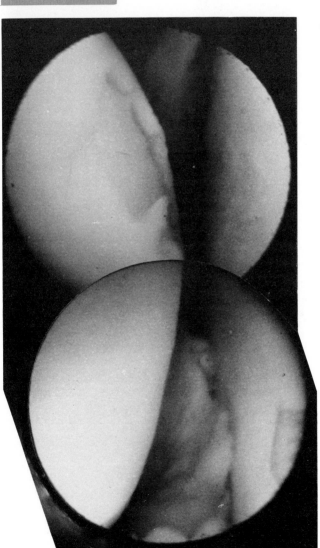

Fig. 4-37. Composite showing retained posterior horn fragment (*left*) and condylar erosion (*right*). In full extension of the knee, the two lesions were in contact.

Chondral and Osteochondral Fractures

In articular cartilage, minor trauma can produce fractures that are not deep enough to involve the underlying bone (Fig. 4-38). These chondral flaps or fractures (Fig. 4-39) can mimic a torn meniscus, blocking the range of motion of a joint and producing a sensation of giving way due to impingement against the intact underlying menisci. As the underlying bone is not involved, these lesions do not show on x-ray. If the cartilage fragment is detached, it becomes a loose body and may leave a characteristic defect at the donor site that can often be identified at arthroscopy (Fig. 4-40, see Plate 10). The edges of the loose fragment are soon rounded, and the fragment becomes a free-floating body (Fig. 4-41), which may continue to cause the knee to buckle. Occasionally, such a fragment retires to a far corner of the joint and becomes attached to the synovium, thereby ending its mischievous activities. This type of cartilage fragment can sometimes be identified and removed through the arthoscope.

If the fracture is deeper and involves subchondral bone, an osteochondral fragment is produced and can often be identified by plain radiography. When the underlying bone is involved, there is always hemorrhage into the joint.

An acute dislocation of the patella usually leaves a sign of the dislocation in the form of a chondral fracture (Fig. 4-42), either of the patella or of the edge of the lateral femoral condyle. Recurrent dislocations usually cause fairly widespread chondromalacia of the patella. The presence of such chondral lesions of the patella or femoral condyle often helps to establish the diagnosis of patellar dislocation or instability.

Osteochondritis Dissecans

Although the articular cartilage overlying areas of osteochondritis dissecans is seldom fibrillated (Fig. 4-43), such lesions may be recognized at

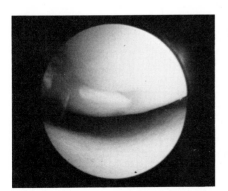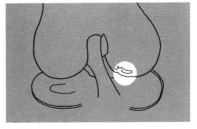

Fig. 4-38.   Small chondral fracture, medial femoral condyle.

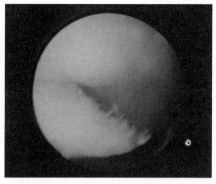 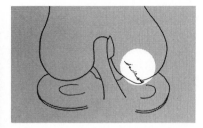

Fig. 4-39.   Triangular chondral fracture of medial femoral condyle limiting extension of the knee. Clinically diagnosed as a torn meniscus.

arthroscopy by actual softening or indentation of the articular cartilage when palpated with the tip of the scope or an examining needle. Occasionally, a split in the cartilage can be explored with the probing needle.

If a fragment of bone or cartilage affected by osteochondritis dissecans is not loose in its bed, we do not operate on it. If arthroscopy shows it to be loose, an operation to remove or secure the fragment is indicated.

Chondromalacia

Fibrillation is the earliest sign of articular cartilage degeneration, and it may be seen on femoral condyles as well as patellae. It is easily recognizable at arthroscopy because the fronds of fibrillated cartilage wave in the "breeze" of the irrigating solution. On an arthroscopic scale of degeneration, this fibrillation would indicate a grade I lesion (Fig. 4-44, see Plate 11). The

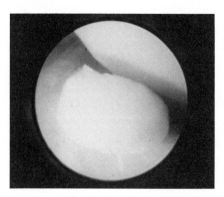 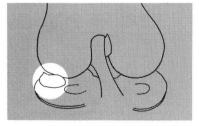

Fig. 4-41.   Cartilaginous loose body in lateral compartment.

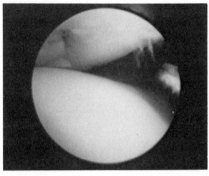
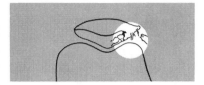

Fig. 4-42.   Recent traumatic dislocation of patella with damage to the articular surface
of the patella.

next stage in the degeneration process, grade II (Fig. 4-45, see Plate 11) is
fragmentation. Large fragments of articular cartilage separate, producing ero-
sions on the articular surface. At this stage, the degenerative process may still
be reversible; but there is no hope of improvement when the next stage, grade
III, is reached, which is essentially complete loss of the hyaline cartilage (Fig.
4-46, see Plate 11). In grade III degeneration the articular surface is yellowish
instead of white and is distinctly irregular or rippled. Osteoarthritis is then well
advanced, and eburnation of the underlying subchondral bone is likely to
follow. Both sides of an articulating joint are usually involved in the degenerative process by the time a grade III lesion is seen.

Although these degenerative changes are most apparent on the patella,
similar changes may be present on the femoral condyles. We see no reason to
consider chondromalacia of the patella as a separate disease process and prefer
to regard it as a result of some other underlying cause, such as malalignment of
the extensor mechanism of the knee. Treatment should be directed primarily

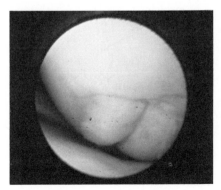
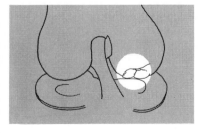

Fig. 4-43.   Osteochondritis dissecans involving medial femoral condyle.

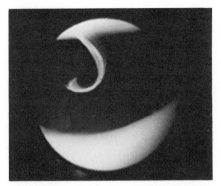 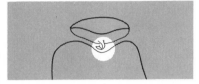

Fig. 4-47. Iatrogenic chondromalacia patella. Articular cartilage damage such as scoring or scraping may occur with forceful insertions of the arthroscope.

toward the cause, not the effect, and should be instituted early, before the irreversible stage of cartilage degeneration is reached. Occasionally, iatrogenic damage to articular cartilage is seen due to scoring or scraping at the time of insertion of the instrument (Fig. 4-47).

Steroid Arthropathy

Subchondral bone resorption can occur after prolonged administration of systemic steroids in the large doses required to suppress the immune response. The articular cartilage sometimes remains intact over a bony defect and can be popped in and out like a dent in a table tennis ball.

Intra-articular steroid injections may be followed by localized but severe fibrillation of the articular cartilage (Fig. 4-48). We have seen this appearance many times and believe that intra-articular steroid injections should be avoided.

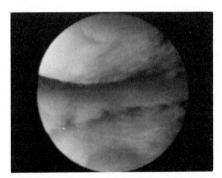 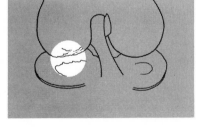

Fig. 4-48. Degenerative changes in both meniscal and articular cartilage are believed to be associated with repeated intra-articular injections of steroid.

CAPSULE AND LIGAMENTS

Anterior Cruciate Ligament

The cruciate ligament can be seen in almost every knee, but its integrity is often difficult to interpret. The ligament is covered with synovium that sometimes masks an incomplete tear, and its insertion is usually so close to the lens that the magnification factor makes abnormalities difficult to assess accurately. Moreover, hypertrophied fat pads or synovial fronds in the anterior part of the joint frequently interfere with visualization.

Despite these problems, enough of the cruciate can usually be seen to determine its integrity (Fig. 4-49, see Plate 12). If complete rupture has occurred, the frayed, tattered, moplike ends of the torn cruciate ligament can easily be identified and the site of rupture determined (Fig. 4-50, see Plate 12). If the ligament is avulsed distally, a plug of bone is usually attached (Fig. 4-51, see Plate 12). With an incomplete tear or a lesion in continuity, the synovium may remain intact, but subsynovial hemorrhagic areas will be seen (Fig. 4-52, see Plate 13). The arthroscopic findings should be evaluated in conjunction with the history of the mechanism of injury and a careful examination of the stability of the knee under general anesthesia.

There is no doubt in our mind that a torn anterior cruciate can exist as an isolated lesion, or at least as the only major abnormality, and closely mimics a torn meniscus. The anterior cruciate usually ruptures in conjunction with varying degrees of capsular disruption, torn menisci, or tears in the collateral ligaments; but again, we prefer to think of a spectrum of ligamentous defects, with complete dislocation of the knee at one end and an isolated anterior cruciate lesion at the other.

Old tears of the anterior cruciate are recognized easily. The proximal end of the distal fragment is rounded, and the enveloping synovial membrane is often absent (Fig. 4-53, see Plate 13). The distal fragment of ligament sometimes causes a feeling of instability, or even a clicking sensation, if it is caught between the weight-bearing areas of the joint. For this reason some surgeons advocate excising the distal end, even as primary treatment, in a tear of the midportion of the anterior cruciate.

Posterior Cruciate Ligament

The bulk of the posterior cruciate ligament cannot be seen with a straight-ahead arthroscope if the anterior cruciate is intact. All that is normally visible is the origin, on the medial femoral condyle, just above the anterior cruciate, covered with synovium and a small amount of fat (Fig. 4-54, see Plate 13). If the anterior cruciate is torn, however, the entire length of the posterior cruciate may be exposed. An old tear of the anterior cruciate with rounded ends gives a particularly good view (Fig. 4-55, see Plate 14).

The tibial attachment of the posterior cruciate may sometimes be seen if a posteromedial approach to the joint is used.

Medial Collateral Ligament

The medial collateral ligament cannot be seen because it is extrasynovial and therefore outside the joint. However, if the ligament has been disrupted from its tibial attachment, a valgus strain will open the medial compartment so that the medial meniscus may appear to float in mid air (Fig. 4-24). A proximal disruption of the ligament tends to leave the meniscus resting on the tibial plateau when a valgus strain is applied.

A rent in the synovium deep to the medial collateral ligament is sometimes visible in cases of recent ligament disruption. In severely disrupted knees, the irrigating solution may escape through such a rent in the synovium and capsule and drain into the subcutaneous tissues to cause massive, but transient, swelling of the calf. A capsular tear should be suspected if joint distension cannot be maintained with the irrigating fluid.

Lateral Collateral Ligament

Laxity of the lateral collateral ligament can be identified at arthroscopy by increased widening of the lateral space. Normally, the posterior horn of the lateral meniscus can be seen easily if a varus strain is applied with the knee in slight flexion. However, in the presence of a lateral tear, the lateral compartment opens much more widely, and the popliteus tendon is demonstrated easily (Fig. 3-16).

Popliteus Tendon

Before arthroscopy was available, the only recognizable abnormality involving the popliteus was accidental division of the tendon during lateral meniscectomy. With arthroscopic examination, however, two other pathological entities can be recognized. Several cases of avulsion of the origin of the popliteus from the femur have been encountered, all occurring from a blow to the back of the extended knee. In this condition, a small fragment of bone attached to the popliteus tendon is avulsed from the point of insertion on the lateral femoral condyle and is pulled into the joint. Hemarthrosis results, with pain in the lateral compartment. Radiological examination shows the small bone fragment in the slightly oblique view. Arthroscopy reveals the fragment of bone attached to its tendon and lying in the lateral gutter (Fig. 4-56, see Plate 14). The recommended treatment is immediate operation and reattachment of the fragment.

Popliteus tendonitis can also be recognized by inflammation of the synovium surrounding the intra-articular portion of the tendon.

Attrition of the Anterior Cruciate Ligament

In the knees of a few patients who have undergone medial meniscectomy, we have observed direct contact between the intact anterior cruciate and the medial border of the lateral femoral condyle as the knee "screws home" in full extension. This contact leads to attrition of the anterior cruciate, and on occasion we have been able to relieve the symptoms by excising bone from the lateral femoral condyle in an attempt to widen the intercondylar notch.

5
The Problems

TECHNICAL PROBLEMS

Adhesions

If synovial adhesions are present, it may be difficult to move the scope within the joint. Often these adhesions can be broken, giving some therapeutic benefit to the patient. The initial distention of the joint often breaks the smaller adhesions and is signalled by a fine popping sensation as the pressure within the joint increases. Stouter adhesions can be broken with the tip of the irrigating needle or even by small scissors inserted through a second sheath.

Adhesions that impede movement into the medial compartment can be broken by replacing the light and telescope with the blunt obturator and sweeping the instrument across the adhesions with controlled force.

Care should be taken not to bend the arthroscope during this maneuver, and one should be aware that the adhesions may be stronger than the instrument. The obturator instead of the telescope should always be inserted for such a maneuver (Fig. 5-1).

The breaking of adhesions invariably causes hemorrhage, and tourniquet control is often necessary (see section on control of bleeding).

Exuberant Synovium

In patients with post-traumatic or inflammatory synovitis, the synovial fronds may be so hyperemic that even gentle movement of the scope can cause

65

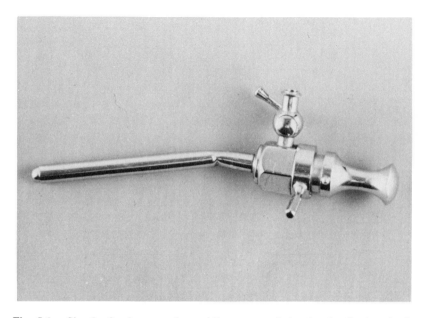

Fig. 5-1.   Sheath of arthroscope bent while surgeon tried to break adhesions in the
medial compartment.

hemorrhage that obscures vision. When this occurs, the tourniquet should be
inflated.

If exuberant synovium engulfs the lens and the surgeon is unable to find
any landmarks within the joint, patience is required. Manipulating the arthroscope at such a time is something like flying above the clouds when the ground
cannot be seen. The tip of the scope is moved cautiously until a break in the
synovial ''cloud'' is seen. One then ''flies'' gently down through the gap to the
white articular cartilage or meniscus beneath. Once the tip of the scope has
negotiated the synovial cumulus, the rest of the examination can proceed
without too much difficulty.

If a single synovial frond obscures vision, it can sometimes be swept out of
the way by the bulb at the tip of the Watanabe 21 arthroscope. Gentle rotation of
the scope is all that is needed.

Subsynovial Space

The beginner may occasionally experience a ''red-out'' in which every-
thing becomes red or reddish orange (or whitish, if the tourniquet is inflated),
and nothing can be identified. This usually means that the tip of the arthroscope
and the light carrier are in the subsynovial space. The instrument has been

withdrawn too far, and the irrigating stream of saline has dissected a small space between the synovium and the underlying fat pad, into which the tip of the scope has fallen. When this occurs, it is best to remove the scope and light carrier, insert the blunt obturator, maneuver the scope back into the suprapatellar pouch, and start again.

A similar appearance might be produced if the saline inflow is blocked or accidently turned off. The joint is then deflated and synovium collapses over the lens, obscuring vision. Reinflation of the joint with saline restores "normality."

Also, saline intended to distend the joint can be injected directly into the subsynovial space. As much as 75 cc can be injected erroneously, thus collapsing the joint space. This problem is avoided if one makes sure that the tip of the needle is in the joint cavity before injecting any saline.

Bleeding

If blood or debris obscures vision and thorough irrigation does not produce a clear field, the tourniquet should be inflated after elevating the leg for 2 minutes. The joint can then be irrigated until clear and the examination continued. At the conclusion of the examination, the tourniquet should be released before the sheath is removed, and the joint should be well irrigated with copious amounts of saline until the efflux is completely clear of blood. It is also wise to irrigate the joint well after a biopsy to minimize any hemorrhage that might have occurred.

Blocked Irrigation and Additional Irrigating Needles

The main outflow needle is frequently blocked by synovial fronds sucked into it by the exit of fluid. This type of blockage can be cleared by gently injecting 5 cc of saline through the needle. Recurrence can be prevented by repositioning the needle so that the bevel points upward and away from the fronds that are striving to block it.

The irrigating needle can also become blocked when it is squeezed against the femur in the suprapatellar pouch as the knee is flexed. If this occurs, a second needle can be inserted in the medial or lateral compartment. The tip of the arthroscope is placed over the desired point of entry on the synovium so that the light indicates the exact spot for insertion and transilluminates the subcutaneous veins. In this way inadvertent venepuncture can be avoided. The entry of the needle may be watched from inside the joint so that the tip of the needle lies in the best position, which is immediately above the meniscus (Fig. 5-2, see Plate 15).

As well as acting as additional irrigation outlets, these extra needles can be used to move loose bodies or to probe for small clefts or lacerations of the meniscus, and defects or softened areas of articular cartilage. Occasionally, an undisplaced bucket-handle tear or a peripheral detachment of the posterior horn can be identified by displacing the meniscal fragment toward the center of the joint. Information gained from this tactile procedure can be very valuable.

Light Failure

Light failure may be a problem with the Watanabe 21 arthroscope. Failure to obtain light at the start of the examination may be due to corrosion at the end of the electrical cord. This can be overcome by gently scraping the cord terminal with a needle or by moistening the connecting end of the light carrier to produce a better contact.

The post of the light carrier sometimes needs cleaning, and small squares of fine-grit emery paper can be kept sterile and used to remove any corrosion or debris. Occasionally, the problem lies at the connection between the bulb and its socket. On its base the Watanabe 21 bulb has a small wire-spring contact that can be accidently flattened and fail to connect with the light carrier. If this occurs, the contact should be teased out or the bulb replaced. If none of these measures are successful, the light carrier, cord, and bulb should each be replaced in turn until the problem is finally corrected. Problems with corrosion may be minimized by proper handling of the instrument and by thorough washing and drying of the arthroscope before sterilization.

Fiber light instruments are less troublesome, but the light source may fail and the user should have on hand ample spare bulbs and fuses.

Finally, the only sure way to avoid cancelling an examination because of instrument failure after the patient has been anesthetized is to keep a second set of equipment sterile and available.

If the Watanabe 21 arthroscope is used too forcefully or if the examiner is not careful, the bulb at the end of the light carrier may catch on a plica or adhesion and bend away from the telescope (Fig. 5-3). This weakens the junction at the tip of the light carrier, and subsequent movements of the scope may cause the bulb to break inside the joint. Therefore, it is wise to lead with the bulb when sweeping inside the joint, so that any obstruction will press the bulb against the telescope, thus preventing bending.

If the light suddenly fails in the middle of an examination, freeze. Do not move the knee or the scope. First, check all external connections, and if these are in order, carefully dismantle the scope and determine whether the bulb or light carrier is broken. If either is broken (and the odds are estimated at 50,000 to 1 against this happening), the knee should be opened immediately and the detached "foreign body" removed. If the position of the knee is not changed, the offending fragment can be located easily.

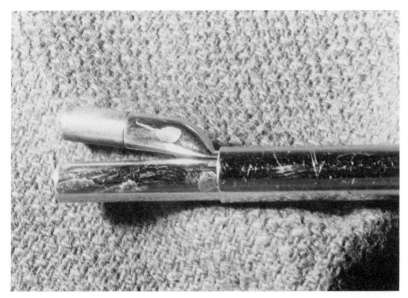

Fig. 5-3.   Bent tip of light carrier, Watanabe 21 (cf Fig. 2-4). This problem should be suspected if visual field becomes dim. Care and gentleness are essential in moving any arthroscope within the knee joint.

DIAGNOSTIC ERRORS

In approximately one-half of the knees that are examined arthroscopically, pathology that is amenable to surgical treatment is found. In these cases, the arthroscopic diagnosis can be confirmed or corrected at the time of arthrotomy. The other cases never come to surgery, so the arthroscopic diagnosis must remain a valid diagnosis until the passage of time or the development of other circumstances provides additional information.

Therefore, in discussing diagnostic accuracy, we can cite only proven errors and must assume that in all other instances the diagnosis is correct until proven otherwise.

As there is always merit in examining one's errors, we shall consider the false diagnoses encountered to date in a consecutive series of 800 cases.

FALSE INTERPRETATIONS

To the best of our knowledge, there have been 5 false-positive interpretations and 6 false-negative interpretations in 800 examinations, for a total of 1.4 percent of cases in which a diagnostic error was made.

In all 5 false-positive patients, arthrotomy would probably have been performed on the basis of clinical assessment, even if arthroscopy had not been available. A surgically amenable abnormality, other than that diagnosed at arthroscopy, was discovered at arthrotomy in 3 of the 5 cases.

In the fourth instance, a normal meniscus was unfortunately removed. The patient's history was typical of a meniscal injury, and the arthrogram was also incorrectly positive. The false-positive arthroscopic interpretation occurred when a large mass of fibrin lying in front of the meniscus was mistaken for a meniscal flap (Fig. 5-4, see Plate 15). The fibrin mass probably resulted from arthrography 3 days previously. To avoid such artifacts, we have discontinued routine arthrography before arthroscopy.

In the fifth false-positive interpretation, a frayed meniscus was removed but no tear was found. This error of interpretation resulted from overestimating the size of small tears in the meniscus due to the magnification of the lens. Both these significant errors occurred in the first 300 cases.

In the 6 false-negative interpretations, a torn meniscus was found on repeat arthroscopy in 3 cases. In these 3 patients, meniscectomy was delayed from 1–9 months as a result of the initially incorrect interpretation. In a fourth patient, the clinical evidence of a torn meniscus was so strong that arthrotomy was undertaken despite the negative findings at arthroscopy, and a meniscal tear was found. In a fifth patient, an exploratory arthrotomy was undertaken because of continuous symptoms, and a rare synovial arteriovenous malformation was found in the suprapatellar pouch. This small lesion had not been recognized at arthroscopy. The sixth patient had several loose bodies that were seen at arthroscopy, but a torn meniscus was also identified at arthrotomy which was not seen arthroscopically.

COMPLICATIONS

There were no instances of infection after arthroscopy alone, but there were four superficial infections and one deep infection in 460 arthrotomies that followed arthroscopy. This represents an incidence of 1.1 percent operative infection rate, which is close to the average for our hospital.

Two patients had transient symptoms of infrapatellar anesthesia after arthroscopy from the anteromedial approach, presumably as a result of damage to the infrapatellar branch of the saphenous nerve at the time of arthroscope insertion.

The bulb of the Watanabe 21 arthroscope broke in a patient who had a torn meniscus, and the fragments were removed at arthrotomy along with the meniscus. This was the only instance of serious equipment failure in 800 cases, although the light carrier was bent on several occasions through rough handling (Fig. 5-3).

In 2 other patients a short circuit from the light carrier (7 volts) caused a tetanic contraction of the quadriceps muscle, which did not result in any discernible after-effects.

There were no instances of thrombophlebitis and no synovial fluid fistulae.

In summary, the complications of arthroscopy are minimal and are probably no greater than those encountered after arthropuncture for any reason.

6

Applications of Arthroscopy

Originally, the arthroscope was considered to be most useful in dealing with "problem" knees. However, with increasing experience, we have found it useful in most knee problems. Knees that are severely disrupted by trauma or disease can, of course, be adequately treated without a preliminary arthroscopic examination, as can knees that have minimal problems, such as minor sprains or contusions. However, between these two extremes are a large number of knee problems that we believe can be better managed by a preliminary endoscopic examination.

Because the morbidity associated with arthroscopy is so minimal, we have developed an aggressive attitude toward establishing a definitive diagnosis as soon as possible after the onset of symptoms. We feel this should be tempered by a conservative attitude toward treatment. Based on this philosophy, the following pages present an overview of how we believe arthroscopy can be useful in managing common knee problems. Although arthroscopy cannot make up for clinical ineptitude, we feel the good clinician becomes even better with this added diagnostic skill.

TRAUMATIZED KNEES

Acute Problems

If a knee has been grossly disrupted by trauma and requires surgical repair because of obvious ligamentous instability, arthroscopy is of little value since the knee will be widely exposed at the time of repair. However, if the injuries are less severe, arthroscopy can provide information about whether the problem might be treated conservatively, or if by doing so an inevitable surgical procedure is merely being delayed.

Most patients with injured knees show symptoms and signs suggesting an internal derangement. In the first few days after injury, it may be difficult to determine whether one or more of the structures inside the knee have been damaged significantly, and, consequently, whether to explore the knee. Many surgeons elect to splint the joint and wait a few days or weeks until "the smoke clears," when persistent symptoms and signs may make the diagnosis more obvious. The availability of arthroscopy has enabled us to determine immediately the condition of the menisci and other intra-articular structures. Also, irrigation removes hemorrhagic material and inflammatory debris, which we believe helps minimize the recovery time of the knees that are subsequently treated conservatively (Fig. 5-2). Even those patients with a meniscal injury that is obvious on clinical assessment may be found at arthroscopy to have one of the other pathological conditions that can mimic a torn meniscus and surgery may be altered or even obviated entirely. In some instances, open operation can also be avoided by corrective intra-articular surgery performed through the arthroscope.

"Million Dollar" Knees

The "million dollar" knee is an exaggerated manifestation of the acutely injured knee and is seen mainly in professional athletes. Large financial decisions often depend on an accurate prognosis of future knee function, and the athlete and his employer are usually unwilling and sometimes unable to wait several weeks to discover the outcome of an injury. The athlete who has sustained a moderate twisting injury (one not severe enough to cause ligamentous instability) which is followed by an effusion can be examined within a few hours or days of the injury; he can then be treated by definitive surgery if indicated, or assured that there is no serious joint defect. With information provided by arthroscopy, the surgeon can plan an effective rehabilitation program, usually shortening the time required for return to normal activity.

Arthroscopy is of value in more ways than just aiding rapid diagnosis in acute athletic injuries. During the off-season, athletes who have had previous injuries or who have undergone knee surgery may seriously consider their future participation in sports. Arthroscopy can provide many answers to questions that were previously unanswerable.

Naturally, professional athletes are not the only individuals with "million dollar" knees. Physical education teachers, high school and college athletes, dancers, and those in less strenuous pursuits but who are on their feet most of the day often wish to know the present state and future prospects of their knee so that they can make career-affecting decisions.

Chronic Problems

Some surgeons may have never removed a normal meniscus in error. Such individuals will find little use for the arthroscope and may not be too tolerant of the frailties of their colleagues. However, we believe that most clinicians are not infrequently in doubt about the diagnosis of a knee that has a history suggestive of a derangement yet little clinical and radiological evidence of such. If the diagnosis is in doubt, arthroscopy can be valuable.

But even when the clinical signs and symptoms are convincingly diagnostic and surgery is planned, we feel that a preoperative arthroscopic examination can be helpful. For example, in 154 consecutive meniscectomies, we found the lesion in the opposite meniscus to that which was clinically suspected in 10 instances (6 percent). Naturally, our surgical approach was altered. If a patient has a suitable injury, followed by a springy block to full extension, an effusion, and localized joint line tenderness, one might argue that there is no need for arthroscopy to confirm the diagnosis of a torn and displaced meniscus. On one hand, we concur with this view because the joint will need to be opened in any event. However, preoperative arthroscopy permits thorough examination of the patellofemoral joint, the other meniscus, and the articular cartilage in the opposite compartment—areas that may be difficult to view completely without a wide incision at meniscectomy.

Some patients with trapped synovium, dislocating anterior horns of menisci, osteochondral and chondral fractures, osteochondritis dissecans, loose bodies, and anterior cruciate injuries may undergo needless meniscectomies if arthroscopy is not undertaken before arthrotomy. Furthermore, some patients have small flaplike or bucket-handle meniscal tears that can be removed through the arthroscope with minimal morbidity. Such patients can be discharged on the day of operation and return to full activity shortly after the procedure (Fig. 6-1).

Use of the Arthroscope in Open Joints

Although the indications are relatively few, arthroscopy can be useful in joints that are already open. The small-diameter fiberscopes enable the surgeon to obtain a better view of the other compartment or the posterior horn region through a limited arthrotomy incision. Extra care should be taken to avoid contamination of the scope by eyebrows or spectacles when the joint is open.

Relationship of Arthroscopy to Arthrography

If both arthroscopy and arthrography are available, the former is the technique of choice. We believe that a routine arthroscopic examination is more valuable than a routine arthrographic examination. The accuracy of diagnosis of meniscal pathology is equally high with either technique, provided a skilled

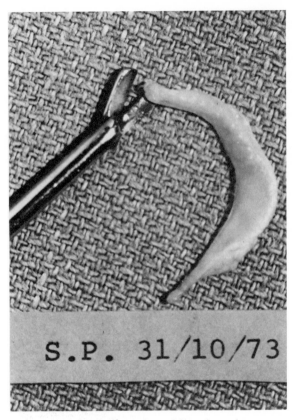

Fig. 6-1. Bucket-handle portion of lateral meniscus removed through the arthroscope after dividing the anterior and posterior attachments with the small scissors.

person is performing the examination. At arthroscopy, however, the menisci can be adequately examined and articular cartilage, synovium, and ligaments—structures that are difficult to interpret radiographically—can be assessed as well. Moreover, should an abnormality be encountered, the arthroscopist—if he is a surgeon—can proceed immediately with corrective measures.

If the arthroscopist has trouble arriving at a diagnosis, arthrography (double contrast is preferred) should be carried out to show specifically the posteromedial corner of the joint.

When arthrography is used as a screening procedure for meniscal derangements, we recommend a delay of at least 7–10 days before performing arthroscopy because the chemical synovitis induced by the contrast medium may affect the visual examination adversely (Fig. 5-4).

ARTHRITIC KNEES

Rheumatoid Arthritis

Rheumatologists will find arthroscopy useful in examining the interior of inflamed knees that defy accurate diagnosis by clinical methods. Arthroscopy of the knee can yield as much information as, if not more than, any exploratory arthrotomy because the synovium can be studied in its natural state. Arthroscopic examination also rules out the question of coexistent pathological findings and allows biopsies to be taken from selected areas that show typical defects (Fig. 6-2, see Plate 16).

The arthroscope may also be used to assess the progress of treatment and to gather information on the natural history of the disease.

The correct strategy for managing the chronically inflamed knee can also be determined by arthroscopy. It is generally recognized that synovectomy can be useful in the early stages of rheumatoid arthritis when the synovium is florid and the articular cartilage is intact. On occasion, we find at arthroscopy that the patient's knee has passed beyond the ideal stage, and that the synovium no longer shows the active appearance of a chronic inflammatory arthritis, but exhibits instead the changes of a secondary osteoarthritis. The articular cartilage may also be seen to be extensively damaged, and in these circumstances it is often better to forego synovectomy and proceed with some other method of treatment.

Degenerative Arthritis

Arthroscopic examination yields little valuable information about advanced osteoarthritis of the tibiofemoral or patellofemoral joints. In some cases, however, it is difficult to determine on clinical grounds whether the patient has a meniscal injury which is in addition to, or may be the reason for, the degenerative process. In such circumstances, arthroscopy can be most helpful. Arthroscopy can also help the surgeon determine what operative procedure might be best for the patient. If a high tibial osteotomy is planned in order to transfer body weight to the supposedly "good" compartment of the knee, arthroscopy may reveal that the "good" compartment of the joint is also involved in the degenerative process, albeit at such an early stage that clinical and radiographic examinations do not suggest this. In such patients, if malalignment is not the main problem, it may be wiser to continue with nonoperative management until the symptoms become severe enough to justify replacement arthroplasty. Some surgeons invariably open the knee joint when doing a high tibial osteotomy to conduct a joint debridement. Others prefer to inflict as little damage as possible on a knee that is already disordered, but they would like to know whether there are torn menisci, loose bodies, or other lesions that could be corrected by some intra-articular procedure. Arthroscopy can identify those patients in whom an arthrotomy is indicated, and it will avoid unnecessary additional trauma to those joints that would not be helped by an arthrotomy.

If one believes that altered biomechanical conditions within the joint can lead to an early onset of degenerative arthritis, then it would follow that the early detection and treatment of pathological conditions (e.g., torn menisci) might aid in preventing degenerative arthritis. Arthroscopy can aid immeasurably in making the early diagnosis.

Finally, temporary but beneficial effects in terms of pain relief have been observed after irrigating the arthritic joint, but these are not as yet explained.

Chondrocalcinosis appears to be markedly improved by the irrigation that accompanies an arthroscopic examination. Of course, the improvement is only temporary since nothing is done to correct the underlying pathological process.

"PROBLEM" KNEES

Postmeniscectomy Knee

One of the most difficult diagnostic problems for surgeons is patients who have persistent symptoms after meniscectomy. The symptoms may include clicking, locking, and swelling, and a retained posterior horn fragment is often diagnosed. Uncommon yet not unknown is the tragic sequence of a medial meniscectomy followed by a series of inappropriate surgical procedures to remove a posterior horn fragment, the opposite meniscus and then the patella, and sometimes followed by a high tibial osteotomy, and eventual arthrodesis. Patients with symptoms after meniscectomy caused us to recognize the inaccuracy of our clinical and radiological diagnostic techniques.

In 174 consecutive arthroscopies referred for diagnosis due to persistent problems after meniscectomy, our diagnosis based on clinical and radiographic examination was accurate in only 58 percent of cases (Fig. 6-3). Arthroscopy revealed that chondromalacia of the femoral condyle was by far the most common diagnosis and was much more common that we had expected (55 percent). Retained posterior horn fragments were diagnosed far too often, and we feel that a symptomatic fragment is a comparatively rare condition (13 percent). Lesions of the opposite meniscus were even rarer and accounted for symptoms in only 5 percent of our cases. Other conditions, including post-traumatic synovitis, chondral fractures, loose bodies, and even early rheumatoid arthritis, were found as unexpected conditions in patients who had undergone meniscectomy. We feel that, especially in this group of patients, the

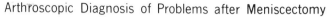

Clinical Versus

Arthroscopic Diagnosis of Problems after Meniscectomy

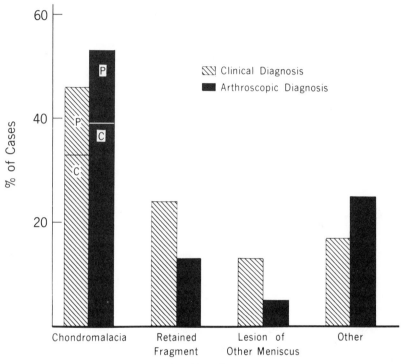

Fig. 6-3.   See text.

use of the arthroscope can avoid many needless arthrotomies in already abnormal knees and can thus significantly reduce future morbidity.

In some instances, further surgery can offer little, and patients must be advised to accept their loss and learn to live with their disability.

Compensation Knee

A comparatively uncommon but particularly valuable indication for arthroscopy arises when a patient is in dispute with his compensation board or insurance company. Such patients are usually persistent and aggressive in their complaints, even though the knee may appear completely normal upon clinical examination. If an exploratory arthrotomy fails to explain the symptoms in such cases, the patients almost always complain of increased discomfort, which from then on might be attributed to the exploratory operation rather than to the original injury. Consequently, most clinicians are reluctant to explore the knees of such patients surgically.

Such individuals need not be outright hysterics or malingerers. Complaining of a persistent knee problem may be a subconscious means of securing attention, a form of secondary gain unrelated to financial aspects. Unfortunately, physicians tend to suspect the motives of patients with troublesome complaints that are inconsistent, inexplicable, and not severe enough to justify arthrotomy.

However, in a study of 186 such patients who were thought to have no knee abnormality, we found a treatable condition in 42 cases (23 percent). In the remaining patients, the clinical impression of normality was confirmed, allowing all parties involved to be firmly reassured of this fact.

Adolescent Knee

Sometimes an adolescent complains of vague symptoms, such as aching, swelling, or giving way, which interfere with schooling and social and athletic pursuits. The patient often is a young girl and is usually seen with her mother, who is more convinced of the severity of the symptoms than the patient is herself. Often the symptoms are attributed to subluxation of the patella with subsequent chondromalacia. At arthroscopy, however, most have no identifiable abnormality and in these instances the physician can reassure the patient and her mother that there is no serious abnormality within the knee. Moreover, this reassurance can be given without scarring the knee or the psyche. Occasionally, an abnormality is found, which is of course a bonus.

Childhood Knee

Although there may be few indications for arthroscopy in the early years of life, the examination probably offers greater potential benefit for children than for adults. We all know that a meniscus can be torn in childhood, even though it is relatively rare. We also know that serious complications may arise 10–15 years later due to the degenerative changes that are precipitated by unrecognized meniscal derangements. Therefore, one must be absolutely certain of the diagnosis before removing a child's meniscus. Moreover, it is advisable to make the diagnosis as soon as possible after the onset of symptoms.

Fortunately, this reliable diagnostic tool, which carries with it little morbidity, is becoming more commonplace. Children above the age of 6 can be examined easily with the larger arthroscopes; smaller instruments must be used for children under 6.

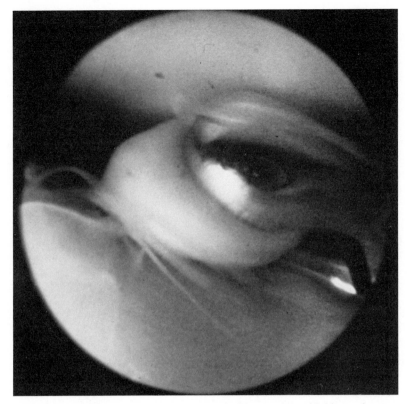

Fig. 6-4.   Small loose body being removed after grasping with biopsy forceps.

Septic Knee

We have had some success in treating acute septic joints by breaking down fibrous adhesions and loculations, irrigating pus from the joint, and establishing drainage and irrigation tubes for subsequent management using the distention-irrigation method described elsewhere.

RESEARCH AND FOLLOW-UP STUDIES

Although it would be difficult to convince a patient to undergo an arthrotomy for research purposes, it is not difficult to secure consent for an arthroscopic evaluation. Consequently, if a patient's other knee is to be examined or he is scheduled for an unrelated surgical procedure requiring anesthesia, a repeat arthroscopic examination can be performed (with informed consent, of course) on the previously treated knee. We have done this in several

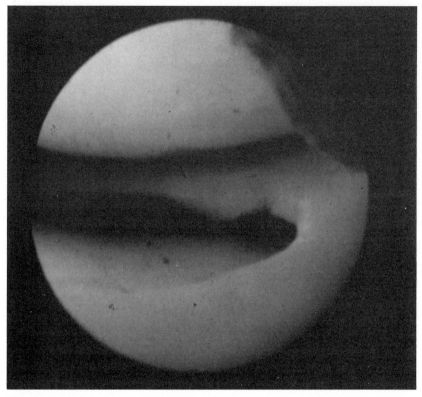

Fig. 6-5.   Medial meniscus immediately after a partial meniscectomy and removal of a small flap.

patients who have undergone shaving procedures, synovectomy, and meniscectomy.

Accurate recordings of the findings at the initial and repeat examinations have enabled us to show interesting but previously undocumented facts about the progress of common conditions. For example, we have documented more accurately than ever before the adverse effects of deranged menisci and meniscectomy on the articular cartilage of the femoral condyles. We have also identified new entities (such as avulsion of the popliteus tendon insertion) and shed light on old problems (such as dislocating menisci). Thus, arthroscopy is in a unique position to contribute significantly to our knowledge of joint pathology and to the effectiveness of treatment.

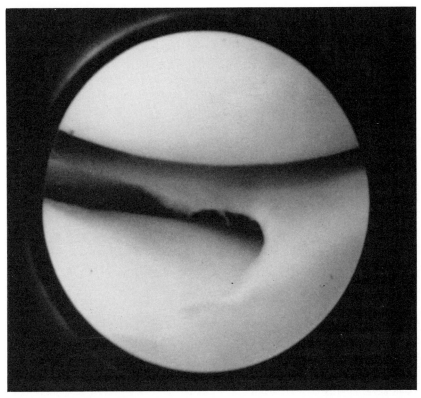

Fig. 6-6.   Appearance of same area (cf Fig. 6-5) 5 years later. Note healthy articular cartilage.

INTRA-ARTICULAR SURGERY

Performing a meniscectomy through the arthroscope is an attractive concept and is a definite possibility in the near future.

Although current techniques are limited, they are no less useful. Small loose bodies can be removed easily through the arthroscope if a firm grasp can be obtained with biopsy forceps (Fig. 6-4).

Transfixing pins have been inserted in loose osteochondral fragments and later removed under direct vision.

Biopsies can be made with precision and with considerably less trauma than that caused by arthrotomy (Fig. 6-2).

Meniscal tags are often small enough to remove through the scope with excellent results. We have also been able to remove displaced bucket handles through the arthroscope (Fig. 6-1) using the small operating scissors included with the Watanabe range of instruments. Alternatively, a small tenotome or even a large hypodermic needle can be passed through the skin and its sharp cutting tip used to divide the fragment from the main body of the meniscus. Figure 4-28 shows a small meniscal tear that was removed through the arthroscope. The immediate postoperative state (Fig. 6-5) can be compared with the appearance 5 years later when the patient was completely free of symptoms (Fig. 6-6). Note the lack of degeneration of articular cartilage on the femoral condyle. Arthroscopy on this occasion was possible because the patient had symptoms in the opposite knee which also warranted arthroscopy, and the follow-up examination was done under the same anesthetic.

On occasion, we have attempted to debride areas of chondromalacia patellae but have not found debridement successful. Stout adhesions in the suprapatellar pouch, the result of trauma or previous surgery, may be broken down by the arthroscope after replacing the telescope and light with the blunt obturator. If the adhesions are particularly thick, they may be divided under direct vision with scissors or a sharp needle. We have also unsuccessfully attempted on one or two occasions to remove remnants of old anterior cruciate tears from the intercondylar notch. Because we could not grasp these structures adequately with the existing forceps, we had to open the joint to achieve successful debridement.

Once we reduced an avulsed tibial spine (Fig. 4-51) by percutaneous manipulation and held it in that position while a cylinder cast was applied. The bone fragment healed strongly and the result was good.

Despite the current limitations of instruments, the possibilities of intra-articular surgery are exciting. Technical advances will doubtless be made in the future, and we look forward to the time when it will be possible to remove entire menisci through a 4-mm incision and discharge the patient the same day to resume his full normal activities.

ARTHROSCOPY IN OTHER JOINTS

The experienced arthroscopist will eventually be drawn toward applying the technique to other joints. It is beyond the scope of this text to outline in any detail the technique of arthroscopy in other joints, but we feel that it is worthwhile to indicate briefly what experience has already shown.

The shoulder joint can be entered anteriorly, laterally, or posteriorly at the joint line and just below the acromion. The principle of distension followed by joint distraction should be followed to facilitate entry. A smaller scope is advantageous in this joint.

The hip joint can be entered best anteriorly after distension with normal saline. X-ray or image intensification should be used to promote accurate entry of the instrument into the joint, just lateral to the femoral vessels and nerve and directly over the anterior aspect of the head of the femur.

The ankle joint can be entered anteriorly, either medially or laterally. Again, a small scope is an advantage, and maximum distension and distraction must be obtained to gain the best visualization.

The elbow joint, wrist joint, and even the metacarpophalangeal joints can also be explored with small scopes.

CONTRAINDICATIONS

The contraindications of arthroscopy are few and are strictly technical. If there is any risk of sepsis, the examination should be postponed. Ankylosis is a definite contraindication. It is almost impossible to maneuver the arthroscope in a joint that is stiffened by severe adhesions. However, useful information can be obtained in knees that have at least 45° of flexion, and a patient rarely is turned down for arthroscopy because of poor flexion. The ideal knee for arthroscopy has a full range of motion and is large and of normal laxity. In such a knee, the scope can be manipulated easily to all corners of the joint. A small, tight knee can make the examination difficult, and a small scope is often required.

7

The Impact of Arthroscopy

IS THE ARTHROSCOPE USEFUL?

Many feel that the arthroscope is little more than an expensive and time-consuming toy. Many experienced surgeons believe that the only clinical decision to be made in managing the knee is whether to open the joint and that to spend 15 minutes or so splashing about in a darkened operating room before every arthrotomy is an unreasonable expenditure of time and money, as well as a sign of professional ineptitude. Some clinicians even say that if after taking a careful history and examining the joint fully a surgeon cannot determine whether a knee needs to be opened, he should give up his interest in the knee and turn to something less complicated and with a more predictable outcome, such as spinal surgery.

We disagree with these views and believe that the arthroscope has an important place in the management of problem knees and also in the practical management of knee disorders as seen in a regular orthopedic practice. Therefore, we have carefully reviewed a series of cases to answer the following questions:

1.   How often does arthroscopic examination alter the management of the patient?
2.   Is the arthroscope of any use in an unselected orthopedic practice, or is its place confined to research and management of problem knees?
3.   How often is the information obtained by arthroscopy wrong?

We studied 800 consecutive arthroscopies covering a 9-year period

(1965–1974). The 800 arthroscopies were done on 705 knees in 675 patients; in some patients both knees were examined, and some knees were examined more than once. In every case, the diagnosis was recorded after taking a careful history, examining the patient, and studying the radiographs. We feel that the surgeon should make a firm clinical diagnosis before arthroscopy and that he should record this diagnosis and the proposed management. Failure to do this can lead to undue reliance on the arthroscope and resulting atrophy of basic clinical skills.

Many of the patients were referred by other doctors specifically for arthroscopy because they had a difficult or unusual problem; thus, we separated patients coming from routine practices from those with problem knees who were referred by other specialists. Of the 800 cases, 68 percent were referred by other specialists and 32 percent came from the emergency department or from general practitioners and were considered to represent a routine and unselected orthopedic practice.

We divided the patients into two main groups according to the management proposed before arthroscopy—those who would have had an arthrotomy and those who would not. Of the total, 614 cases (77 percent) would have undergone open operation if the arthroscope had not been available. We considered that arthroscopy had no real effect on the treatment or progress of 253 of these (Table 7-1). However, in some of these patients (26 percent), exact knowledge of the abnormality—a loose body or retained posterior horn fragment, for example—allowed the surgeon to use a smaller incision than would otherwise have been possible. In others (24 percent), the clinical diagnosis was proved wrong, or an additional defect was found, but we considered that this discovery did not alter the outcome because the true condition would have been found at arthrotomy. In the remaining cases (50 percent), arthroscopy had no impact on the patients' care. These 253 cases (41 percent of all those that would have undergone arthrotomy) were not significantly helped by arthroscopy, and the critics of the technique would be justified in commenting that the examination was unnecessary and prolonged the duration of the anesthesia.

Table 7-1
Cases in Which Management Was Not Altered after Arthroscopy

Result	Routine Cases	Referred Cases	Total
Clinical diagnosis confirmed	60 (59%)	66 (44%)	126 (50%)
Smaller incision used	16 (16%)	51 (34%)	67 (26%)
Different diagnosis	16 (16%)	24 (16%)	40 (16%)
Additional diagnosis	10 (9%)	10 (6%)	20 (8%)
Total	102 (100%)	151 (100%)	253 (100%)

In the remaining 361 cases (59 percent), the reverse was true, for we consider that the actual management of these patients was directly influenced by the findings of arthroscopy. Open operation was avoided in 196 cases (Table 7-2) because the clinical diagnosis was not confirmed or the condition was not considered amenable to surgery (58 percent), or the arthroscopy was performed merely to rule out an operable lesion (32 percent). In a further 20 knees (10 percent), the operative procedure was done through the arthroscope and arthrotomy was thus avoided altogether. These patients included 6 in whom a loose body was found and removed through the arthroscope and 14 in whom synovial biopsy or a partial meniscectomy was done through the instrument.

We were particularly concerned with 114 patients in whom open operation was cancelled because the arthroscopic examination suggested that the clinical diagnosis was wrong or the abnormality seen was not considered amenable to surgery. We feared that these patients had simply gone elsewhere and undergone operation by another surgeon. We therefore reviewed these patients by personal interview and examination when possible, or by questionnaire. We traced 106 of the 114 patients. The mean interval between arthroscopy and review was 25 months, with a range of 6 months to 7 years. Six of the patients had subsequently undergone operation and were improved by surgery. However, 8 others had also undergone operation elsewhere and stated that they had been made worse. Of the remaining 92 patients, 73 had improved without operation, 2 had become worse, and 16 were unchanged. The remaining patient developed unmistakable signs of insanity and required psychiatric treatment. We concluded from this review that the arthroscopic decision to cancel open operation was justified in 98 out of 106 occasions (93 percent).

In the other 165 of the 361 cases in which operation was strongly influenced by the findings of arthroscopy, the patient either underwent a different operation altogether or the surgical strategy was drastically altered (Table 7-3). The most obviously successful of this group were 27 patients (16 percent) in whom a different diagnosis was made and an entirely different operation performed. In 10 of these, a lesion was found in the meniscus opposite to that originally considered damaged.

In 33 patients (20 percent), an operation was done without opening the joint, which would have been necessary if the arthroscope had not been

Table 7-2

Patients in Whom Open Operation Was Avoided after Arthroscopy

Result	Routine Cases	Referred Cases	Total
Condition not amenable to operation	37	77	114 (58%)
Exploratory arthrotomy avoided	13	49	62 (32%)
Procedure done through arthroscope	5	15	20 (10%)
Total	55	141	196 (100%)

Table 7-3
Modification of Treatment Resulting from Arthroscopy

Result	Routine Cases	Referred Cases	Total
Future strategy planned	24	81	105 (64%)
Joint not opened	13	20	33 (20%)
Different operation done	13	14	27 (16%)
Total	50	115	165 (100%)

available—for example, patients undergoing tibial osteotomy for degenerative arthritis were sometimes thought preoperatively to need joint debridement or meniscectomy, until the arthroscope showed that this was unnecessary. However, the bulk of this group consisted of 105 patients (64 percent) in whom the timing or the nature of operation was determined by arthroscopy. Some of these patients were considered on clinical and radiological grounds to be good candidates for a high tibial osteotomy, as they appeared to have a comparatively healthy compartment to which their body weight could be transferred. However, at arthroscopy it was found that the supposedly healthy compartment was quite severely disorganized, and operation was deferred until the symptoms merited prosthetic replacement.

Of the 800 cases, 186 would have been managed without open operation if the arthroscope had not been available. This group included patients with dramatic or bizarre symptoms that did not correspond to physical signs or history, patients with medicolegal problems, alleged hysterics and malingerers, and high-performance athletes such as ballet dancers and quarterbacks. In 131 of these (70 percent), arthroscopy was helpful only in confirming the clinical impression that open operation was unnecessary. Even though the arthroscopic examination did not alter the eventual management of these patients, it did enable the clinician to reassure the patient with absolute confidence that no operation was needed. On other occasions, professional athletes could be given a rapid and confident judgment on which to base a decision affecting their future careers.

A treatable condition was found unexpectedly in 42 patients (23 percent). This was particularly valuable if the patient had previously been considered a hysteric or a malingerer or had been the subject of medicolegal acrimony. In the remaining 13 patients (7 percent), a procedure such as partial meniscectomy or biopsy was done that would not have been warranted if arthrotomy had been required.

When we began this review, we expected to find that the arthroscope was of special value in the referred problem knees and of little use in a routine orthopedic practice. Not until the final results were analyzed did we discover,

Table 7-4
Overall Effect on Management in 800 Cases

Result	Routine Cases	Referred Cases	Total
Patients who would have undergone arthrotomy (614 cases)			
No difference in management	102 (49%)	151 (37%)	253 (41%)
Open operation avoided	55 (27%)	141 (35%)	196 (32%)
Treatment modified	50 (24%)	115 (28%)	165 (27%)
Total	207 (100%)	407 (100%)	614 (100%)
Diagnostic arthroscopy (186 cases)			
No difference in management	28 (61%)	103 (74%)	131 (70%)
Treatable condition found	14 (30%)	28 (20%)	42 (23%)
Procedure done through arthroscope	4 (9%)	9 (6%)	13 (7%)
Total	46 (100%)	140 (100%)	186 (100%)

with some satisfaction, that the use of the arthroscope resulted in an important difference in management in 51 percent of the patients encountered in a routine orthopedic practice who would have undergone open operation. By the same token, 63 percent of the referred patients were influenced positively by the examination. The figures are less gratifying in the group of patients who would have been managed without operation if the arthroscope had not been available. Nevertheless, 39 percent of routine patients and 26 percent of referred cases derived some positive benefit from arthroscopy. The overall results of the study are outlined in Table 7-4.

From this review, we concluded that arthroscopy is a valuable technique in a routine and uncomplicated orthopedic practice and is almost indispensable to those surgeons with a special interest in the knee who deal with referred problems. However, its usefulness depends to a certain extent on surgical philosophy. Some surgeons can always find a reason for having opened the knee once they have done it, such as an osteophyte to be trimmed, or a hypermobile meniscus to be removed. In contrast, the conservative surgeon who believes the knee to be a cantankerous and irritable joint that takes unkindly to unnecessary meddling will find the arthroscope to be of inestimable value in avoiding needless violation.

Bibliography

1. Amako T: On the injuries of the menisci in the knee joint of Japanese. J Jap Orthop Assoc 33:1289, 1960 (Jap).
2. Andersen RB, Rossel I: Arthroscopy of the knee joint in rheumatic diseases. Ugeskr Laeger 135:71, 1973 (Dan).
3. Bircher E: Die arthroendoskopie. Zentralbl Chir 48:1460–1461, 1921 (Ger).
4. Bircher E: Bietrag aur pathologie (Arthritis deformans) und diagnose der meniscusverletzungen (Arthroendoskopie). Bruns Z Klin Chir 127:239, 1955 (Ger).
5. Burman MS: Arthroscopy or direct visualization of joints. An experimental cadaver study. J Bone Joint Surg 13:669–695, 1931.
6. Burman MS, Finkelstein H, Mayer L: Arthroscopy of the knee joint. J. Bone Joint Surg 16:255–268, 1934.
7. Burman MS, Mayer L: Arthroscopic examination of the knee joint. Arch Surg 32:846, 1936.
8. Burman MS, Sutro CJ: Arthroscopy by fluorescence; experimental study. Arch Phys Therapy 16:423, 1935.
9. Butt WP, McIntyre JL: Double-contrast arthrography of the knee. Radiology 92:487–499, 1969.
10. Casscells SW: Arthroscopy of the knee joint; a review of 150 cases. J Bone Joint Surg 53-A:287–298, 1971.
11. Dandy DJ, Jackson RW: The diagnosis of problems after meniscectomy. J Bone Joint Surg 57-B, 3:349–52, 1975.
12. Dandy DJ, Jackson RW: The impact of arthroscopy on the management of disorders of the knee. J Bone Joint Surg. 57-B, 3:346–48, 1975.

13. Dandy DJ, Jackson RW: Meniscectomy and chondromalacia of the femoral condyles. J Bone Joint Surg. 57-A, 8:116–119, 1975.

14. Dashefsky JH: Discoid lateral meniscus in three members of a family. J Bone Joint Surg (Am) 53:1208, 1971.

15. Delbarre F, Aignan M, Ghozlan R: "L'Arthroscopie du genou". Institut de Rhumatologie de la faculte de medicine de Paris-Cochin. 1975 (Fre).

16. Dorfmann H, de Seze C: Filarial monoarthritis. A propos of a case diagnosed by arthroscopy. Nouv Presse Med 1:1013, 1972 (Fre).

17. Dorfmann H, Dreyfus P: Arthroscopy of the knee (methods and results). Cah Med 12:561, 1971 (Fre).

18. Dorfmann H, Dreyfus P: Arthroscopy of the knee; methods and results. Minerva Med 62:2621, 1971 (It).

19. Dorfmann H, Dreyfus P: Arthroscopy of the knee; methods and results. Rev Clin Esp 121:545, 1971 (Spa).

20. Dorfmann H, Dreyfus P, Justin-Besancon L, et al: Arthroscopy of the knee joint. Current status of the question. Sem Hop Paris 46:3442, 1970 (Fre).

21. Dorfmann H, de Seze S: Nouvelles observations sur l'arthroscopie du genou. Resultat d'une experience personnelle. Sem Hop Paris 48. No. 46:3011–3019, 1972 (Fre).

22. Eikelaar HR: Arthroscopy of the knee—Thesis for a doctorate in orthopaedic surgery at the University of Groningen. The Netherlands, Royal United Printers Hoitsema B.V., 1975.

23. Finkelstein H, Mayer L: The arthroscope, a new method of examining joints. J Bone Joint Surg 13:583–588, 1931.

24. Fujimoto K: Arthroscopic findings of the experimental arthritis caused by intra-articular injection of various disinfectant medicaments. J Jap Orthop Assoc 22:60, 1949 (Jap).

25. Gallannaugh S: Arthroscopy of the knee joint. Br Med J 3:285, 1973.

26. Geist ES: Arthroscopy: preliminary report. Lancet 46:306–307, 1926.

27. Henry A: Arthroscopy of the knee joint. Guys Hosp Rep 121:25, 1972.

28. Hoffa A: The influence of the adipose tissue with regard to the pathology of the knee joint. JAMA 43:795–796, 1904.

29. Huckell JR: Is meniscectomy a benign procedure? A long-term follow-up study. Can J Surg 8:254–260, 1965.

30. Hurter E: L'Arthroscopie, nouvelle methode d'exploration du genou. Rev Chir Orthop 41:763–766, 1955 (Fre).

31. Iino S: Normal arthroscopic findings of the knee joint in adults. J Jap Ortho Assoc 14:467, 1939 (Jap).

32. Imbert R: Arthroscopy; significance of the method. Mars Chir 9:676, 1957 (Fre).

33. Imbert R: Arthroscopy of the knee; its technique. Mars Chir 8:368, 1956 (Fre).

34. Jackson RW, McCarthy DD: Arthroscopy of the knee. *In,* Gordon DE (ed): Proceedings of the Fourth Canadian Conference on Research in the Rheumatic Diseases. Toronto, University of Toronto Press, 1971, p 293–297.

35. Jackson RW, Abe I: The role of arthroscopy in the management of disorders of the knee; an analysis of 200 consecutive examinations. J Bone Joint Surg 54-B:310–322, 1972.

36. Jackson RW: Arthroscopy of the knee. *In,* Ahstrom JP Jr (ed): Current Practice in Orthopaedic Surgery, Vol. 4; 1973, p 93–117.

37. Jackson RW: The role of arthroscopy in the management of the arthritic knee. Clin Orthop 101:28–35, 1974.

38. Jackson RW: Diagnostic uses of arthroscopy. *In,* McKibbin B (ed): Recent Advances in Orthopaedics, Vol. 10, London, Churchill Livingstone, 1975, p 217–234.

39. Jackson RW, DeHaven K: Arthroscopy of the knee. Clin Orthop 107:87, 1975.

40. Jackson RW, Parsons CJ: Distension-irrigation treatment of major joint sepsis. Clin Orthop 96:160–164, 1973.

41. Jayson MIV, Dixon AStJ: Arthroscopy of the knee in rheumatic diseases. Ann Rheum Dis 27:503, 1968.

42. Jayson MIV: Arthroscopy; a new diagnostic method. Nurs Times 64:1002, 1968.

43. Johnson LL: Diagnostic arthroscopy of the knee. Proceedings of the International Congress of the Knee-Joint. Rotterdam, Excerpta Medica Amsterdam, 1973.

44. Kaplan EB: Discoid lateral meniscus of the knee joint; nature, mechanism and operative treatment. J Bone Joint Surg (Am) 39:77, 1957.

45. Kawashima W: Arthroscopy of the tuberculous knee in its early stage. J Jap Orthop Assoc 18:651, 1943 (Jap).

46. Koike F: Arthroscopic study of experimental suppurative arthritis. J Jap Orthop Assoc 18:656, 1943 (Jap).

47. Kreuscher P: Semilunar cartilage disease, a plea for early recognition by means of the arthroscope and early treatment of this condition. Ill Med J 47:290–292, 1925.

48. Lipson RL, Clemmons JJ, Frymoyer JW: Arthroscopy: Experience with percutaneous biopsy of intraarticular structures under direct vision. Arthritis Rheum 10:294, 1967.

49. Marques J, Santamaria A, Gomez Martinez G et al: Arthroscopy. Rev Esp Reum Enferm Osteoartic 14:47, 1971 (Spa).

50. Matsumo J: Arthroscopic and histological studies of tuberculous and
     non-specific chronic arthrtides. J Jap Assoc Rheum 1:409, 1959 (Jap).
51. Mayer, L, Burman MS: Arthroscopy in the diagnosis of meniscal le-
     sions of the knee joint. Am J Surg 43:501, 1939.
52. Mennet P: Potential and limits of knee arthroscopy. Schweiz Med
     Wochenschr 101:1591, 1971 (Ger).
53. Nicholas JA, Freiberger RH, Killoran PJ: Double-contrast arthrog-
     raphy of the knee; its value in the management of 225 knee derange-
     ments. J Bone Joint Surg 52-A:203–220, 1970.
54. O'Connor RL: The arthroscope in the management of crystal-induced
     synovitis of the knee. J Bone Joint Surg 55-A:1443–1449, 1973.
55. O'Connor RL: Arthroscopy in the diagnosis and treatment of acute
     ligament injuries of the knee. J Bone Joint Surg 56-A, 2:333–337,
     1974.
56. Ohnsorge J: Arthroskopie des kniegelenkes mittels Glasfasern. Z Or-
     thop 106:535, 1969 (Ger).
57. Ohnsorge J: Color photography of the inner space of the knee joint
     using a new glass fiber endoscope. Langenbecks Arch Chir 325:965,
     1969 (Ger).
58. Okamura T: An arthroscopic study of the traumatic disorders of the
     knee joint. J Jap Orthop Assoc 23:28, 1945 (Jap).
59. Robles Gil J, Katona G, Barroso MR: Arthroscopy as an aid to diag-
     nosis and investigation. Excerpta Medica International Congress Series
     143:16, 1968.
60. Robles Gil J, Katona G: Arthroscopy as a means of diagnosis and
     research; review of 80 arthroscopies. In, Katona G, Robles Gil J
     (eds): Proceedings of the Fourth Pan American Congress of Rheumatol-
     ogy, Mexico City, 1967. Amsterdam, Excerpta Medica 209, 1969.
61. Robles Gil J, Katona G: Clinical and therapeutic usefulness of arthros-
     copy. Gazz Sanit 20:16, 1971 (It).
62. Sato K: An arthroscopic study of knee joint injury caused by dull force.
     J Jap Orthop Assoc 24:184, 1950 (Jap).
63. Sato K: An arthroscopic study of knee joint injury caused by dull force.
     J Jap Orthop Assoc 28:467, 1955 (Jap).
64. Sommer R: Die endoskopie des kniegelenkes. Zentralbl Chir 64:1692,
     1937 (Ger).
65. Suckert R: Photoarthroscopy of the knee joint. Z Unfallmed Berufskr
     53:65, 1960 (Ger).
66. Takagi K: Practical experience using Takagi's arthroscope. J Jap Or-
     thop Assoc 8:132, 1933 (Jap).
67. Takagi K: The arthroscope. J Jap Orthop Assoc 14:359–441, 1939
     (Jap).

68. Tesson MC, Aignan M, Delbarre F: Arthroscopy of the knee. Technique, indications, results. Presse Med 78:2467, 1970 (Fre).

69. Tsuyama N, Udagawa E: Arthroscopy. Surg Ther (Osaka) 14:581, 1966 (Jap).

70. Vaubel E: Die arthroskopie (Endoskopie des kniegelenkes) eibeitrag zur diagnostiek der gelenkkrankheiten. Zeitschrift fur Rheumaforschung Band 9, 1, 210, 1938 (Ger).

71. Watanabe M: Arthroscopy of the ankle joint of the horse. J Jap Orthop Assoc 22:51, 1949 (Jap).

72. Watanabe M: The development and present status of the arthroscope. J Jap Med Instr 25:11, 1954 (Jap).

73. Watanabe M, Takeda S, Ikeuchi H: Atlas of arthroscopy. Tokyo, Igaku Shoin Ltd., 1957.

74. Watanabe M, Takeda S: The number 21 arthroscope. J Jap Orthop Assoc 34:1041, 1960 (Jap).

75. Watanabe M, Takeda S, Ikeuchi H: Atlas of Arthroscopy (2nd Ed). Tokyo, Igaku Shoin Ltd., 1969.

76. Watanabe M: Arthroscopy of the knee joint. In, Helfet AJ (ed): Disorders of the Knee. New York, J.B. Lippincott, 1974, p 139–149.

77. "From Lichleiter to Fiber Optics"—Catalogue prepared by the staff of the national museum for the history of science, Leiden, the Netherlands, on the occasion of the XVIth Congress of the International Society for Urology.

Index

                                                        a
                                                        b
                                                        c
                                                    6   d
                                                    7   e
                                                    8   f
                                                    9   g
                                                    0   h
                                                    1   i
                                                8   2   j